GABRIELLE KAPLAN-MAYER is a writer, performer, and educator. She is the author of several plays and one-woman shows. A 1993 graduate of Emerson College with a B.F.A. cum laude in performing arts, she also earned a master's degree in Jewish studies at the Reconstructionist Rabbinical College. Gabrielle currently teaches playwriting for the Philadelphia Young Playwrights Festival and is a consultant in the creative arts for the Auerbach Central Agency for Jewish Education. She has had diabetes since she was ten years old and has been on the pump since 1999.

Insulin Pump Therapy Demystified

Insulin Pump Therapy Demystified

AN ESSENTIAL GUIDE
FOR EVERYONE PUMPING INSULIN

Gabrielle Kaplan-Mayer

Foreword by Gary Scheiner, M.S., C.D.E.

MARLOWE & COMPANY ■ NEW YORK

INSULIN PUMP THERAPY DEMYSTIFIED:
An Essential Guide for Everyone Pumping Insulin
Copyright © 2003 by Gabrielle Kaplan-Mayer
Foreword copyright © 2003 by Gary Scheiner, M.S., C.D.E.

Published by
Marlowe & Company
An Imprint of Avalon Publishing Group Incorporated
161 William Street, 16th Floor
New York, NY 10038

Library of Congress Control Number: 2002113886
Library of Congress Cataloging-in-Publication Data is available for this title.

ISBN 1-56924-508-8

9 8 7 6 5 4 3 2 1

Designed by Pauline Neuwirth, Neuwirth & Associates

Printed in the United States of America
Distributed by Publishers Group West

This book is dedicated to all the researchers who have made the dream of insulin pump therapy into a reality, to all the early pump users who were willing to try pump therapy when it was truly in its pioneering stage, and to all the many pump users whose stories have helped me to create this book.

CONTENTS

Foreword by Gary Scheiner, M.S., C.D.E.   xi

Introduction: We're in This Challenge Together!   1

PART ONE: To Pump or Not to Pump?   7

  ONE: What Is an Insulin Pump and   9
Why Would I Want One?

  TWO: Seeking Knowledge   14

  THREE: Finding Support   24

  FOUR: Making the Commitment   31

PART TWO: What's It Really Like to Live with the Pump?   37

  FIVE: Body Image, Fashion, and Visibility   39

  SIX: Sleeping with the Pump   50

  SEVEN: And Now, Ladies and Gentlemen . . .   54
the Question You've All Been Waiting For:
Sex and the Pump!

  EIGHT: Money Makes the World Go Round . . .   60

  NINE: Inconvenience, or How Much More   66
Do I Need to Schlepp?

  TEN: The Mechanics of the Pump, or   71
"But I Can't Even Program My VCR!"

  ELEVEN: Exercise with the Pump   76

TWELVE: Swimming, Water Sports, 84
and Days at the Beach

PART THREE: Preparing to Pump— 89
What You Need to do Before Your "Big Day"

THIRTEEN: Which Pump to Choose? 91

FOURTEEN: Carbohydrate Counting, or 102
What Evil Lies Within That Slice of Pizza?

FIFTEEN: Your First Days on the Pump 112

PART FOUR: Happily Pumping Ever After . . . 119

SIXTEEN: The First Few Weeks 121

SEVENTEEN: Weight Management and the Pump: 126
Watching Those Pounds

EIGHTEEN: Troubleshooting the Bumps in the Road 131

NINETEEN: Your Emotional Health 137

TWENTY: Staying Motivated 143

TWENTY-ONE: Pump Therapy and Travel 148

PART FIVE: Pumping for Everyone! 153
Kids, Teens, Seniors, and Moms-to-Be

TWENTY-TWO: Pumping Kids 155

TWENTY-THREE: Pumping Teens 161

TWENTY-FOUR: Pumping Seniors 166

TWENTY-FIVE: Pumping During Pregnancy 170

EPILOGUE: What Lies Ahead in 176
Insulin Pump Technology

Glossary of Diabetes and Insulin Pump Terms 179
Counting Carbohydrates 181
References 183
Acknowledgments 185
Index

FOREWORD

BACK IN 1984, when home blood glucose monitoring was just beginning to reach the mainstream (my first meter was the size of a sandwich and took two minutes and a pint of blood to give a reading), I was lucky enough to be diagnosed with the "condition" known as type 1 diabetes. Back then, the four magic words were: diet, exercise, insulin, and monitoring. You took your insulin (two shots a day were the norm) and conformed the rest of your life to the peaks and valleys of your insulin program.

Today I run my own practice specializing in intensive diabetes management. The four magic words have been replaced by a simple four-word phrase: THINK LIKE A PANCREAS. It is this mantra by which I teach patients how to self-manage their diabetes. To manage this disease properly, you simply have to know how to match your insulin to your needs. And nothing enables us to THINK LIKE A PANCREAS more than using an insulin pump. Pumps afford us the opportunity to administer boluses of insulin with extreme precision on an as-needed basis. They also allow us to fine-tune the level of basal insulin to match diurnal variations in endogenous glucose production and insulin sensitivity. The result is a combination of improved glycemic control and a freer, more flexible lifestyle.

People of all ages use insulin pumps to match their insulin doses to their precise needs. Momentary adjustments can be made for variations in food intake, physical activity, and emotions. Accommodation can easily be made for fluctuations in hormone production that accompanies events such as illness, growth, puberty, pregnancy, and menopause.

For me, the pump has brought a level of control that I could not achieve with injections. And I'm not talking about HbA1c; mine has not changed much from the time I was on shots to the time I've been on the pump. I'm talking about *quality* blood sugar control: fewer highs and lows, and more readings within my target range.

I enjoy many forms of exercise, from long-distance cycling to boxing to basketball. When I took insulin injections, low blood sugars were common after I worked out. Some were severe enough to require visits to the emergency room. The pump lets me adjust for both the immediate and delayed effects of exercise. In eight years of pump use, I'm proud to report *zero* episodes of severe hypoglycemia.

Meal scheduling was also a challenge with insulin injections. Who can eat all three meals at the same time every day? I no longer have to worry about dropping low if a meal is delayed. Now I can occasionally work through lunch, take my wife out for a late dinner, or miss breakfast to play with the kids, work around the house or (gasp!) even sleep a little late.

Using an insulin pump is by no means simple. It takes adequate preparation, training, and follow-through. Having trained more than five hundred people on insulin pump therapy, the characteristics and skills that I have found to be most valuable are: (1) frequent blood glucose testing; (2) detailed record keeping; (3) good carbohydrate gram counting skills; (4) an ability to self-adjust insulin doses properly; and (5) a true desire to give the pump a try. Very few people are 100 percent convinced that the pump is right for them until they have given it a fair trial period. The first few weeks can be somewhat frustrating. But once you get over the initial mechanical adjustments and start seeing your blood sugars stabilize, you'll be hooked. More than 90 percent of all people who have ever tried an insulin pump are still using an insulin pump. (In my practice, because of the intense education that precedes and follows pump initiation, that number is closer to 99 percent.) In fact, the most common complaint I hear about pump therapy is "I wish I had tried it years ago."

Why, then, are so many people with insulin-dependent diabetes still taking injections? It probably has a lot to do with misinformation. People tend to fear what they do not understand. Physicians are no exception—ask doctors who are unfamiliar with pump therapy, and most will discourage you from using it. Those familiar with it are almost sure to give it the thumbs-up.

It is also a lack of understanding among people with diabetes that has kept the number of pump users so low (approximately 10 percent of those with insulin-dependent diabetes are using pump therapy). That's where this book can be so valuable. Besides the nuts and bolts of what a pump is and how it works, this book delves into the art and science of *living* with an insulin pump. Gabrielle Kaplan-Mayer has done a masterful job of touching on all the "touchy" subjects that deter non-pump users and challenge those new to pump therapy. Everything from insurance issues to concealing the pump in one's clothing to "what to do with it" during sex.

Speaking of sex, I was once delivering a lecture on pump therapy to a group of pharmacy students, and was asked if I could have sex with the pump. I looked the promising young pharmacist right in the eye and responded, "I suppose, but I'd rather have sex with my wife."

Gotta keep a sense of humor about this stuff! Enjoy the book.

Gary Scheiner M.S., C.D.E.
Owner, Integrated Diabetes Services
Wynnewood, Pa.

We're in This Challenge Together!

I WAS DIAGNOSED with juvenile, or type 1, diabetes on January 2, 1982, when I was ten years old. For weeks I had been suffering from typical symptoms—constant thirst, frequent urination, lack of energy. I remember feeling "not quite right" but couldn't articulate what was wrong. I was totally shocked—as was my family—when the results of a urine test proved I had a chronic illness.

When I heard the word "diabetes," all I knew was that it was an illness of some kind and thought it must be serious. I was scared I might die. When I entered the hospital that day, doctors and nurses explained that diabetes was a livable condition, that I'd have to take insulin shots and watch what I ate, but that otherwise I'd be okay. All day long, I kept wondering, "Will I still be able to live a normal life?" From as early as I remember, I wanted to be a mom someday. Would I live a long time with diabetes? Would I be able to do the normal things everyone gets to do? Would I grow up and get to have a family of my own?

Initially, I adapted pretty well to living with diabetes; I practiced giving insulin shots to an orange and injected insulin into my own skin on the second day after I was diagnosed. Back then, the doctors gave me strips to test my urine. Chemstrips were still a few years away. I gave up eating cookies and candy altogether and indulged only in a once-a-week ice cream cone. Despite feeling "different" from my friends who didn't have diabetes, I managed all right for those first few years.

One day (I was maybe twelve years old), I was reading *Diabetes Forecast* magazine. There was an article in it about complications: blindness, kidney failure, retinopathy. I was shocked. No one had ever talked to me about this stuff before! I asked my mom if it was true, that all of these terrible things happened to people with diabetes. She told me that they were working on cures for the complications and that these things wouldn't happen to me. I don't know what else you would tell a child. Still feeling shocked and scared, I didn't know if I should believe her. Over the next few years, technology helped me to improve my care—within four years of my diagnosis, I had a blood sugar meter and better syringes. Research came out saying that tight control helped to prevent complications. My doctors worked with me to teach me how to keep as tight a control—keeping my blood sugars as close to the normal range—as possible.

During my late teen years and the start of college, I became angry at my diabetes and was sick and tired of the work I had to do to keep tight control. I wanted to eat and drink whatever I wanted, just like my friends. I experimented a lot and ignored my diabetes. Caught up in the romance and passion of youth, I decided it was better to "live hard and die young" than to put up with a life of carefully scheduled meals and constant shots and testing. I would go days on end without pricking my finger and would skip meals when I felt like it. Somehow, amazingly, I never got too sick or suffered a severe hypo- or hyperglycemia episode.

By the time I graduated college, my constant rebelling had lost its sexiness and I realized that like it or not, my diabetes was here to stay. I'd have to figure out some way to deal with it if I wanted to pursue my dreams of becoming a writer and getting married and having a family. For the next few years, I tried really hard to work with my diabetes. I saw different doctors. My body was going through some major hormonal changes. I started getting severe premenstrual symptoms seven to ten days before my menstrual cycle: depression, bloating, cramps. Worst of all, my blood sugars would go out of control no matter what I did. I could be 120 one minute, and a few hours later test at 320. I saw this pattern develop month after month. It took visits to several doctors before I found one who believed me and would work with this condition! Still, adding extra shots of regular insulin during those days never quite cut it. I became resigned to feeling simply miserable, physically and emotionally, two weeks out of every month. I imagined the complications that were starting in my body because my sugars were running high. This fear made me even more depressed and tense.

During the two weeks that I wasn't suffering from PMS, I still had trouble with my morning blood sugars. My doctor explained that I had something called the "dawn phenomenon"—during the very early hours of the morning, my blood sugar would rise for no expected reason. We tried working with multiple injection therapy—adjusting my evening NPH insulin and taking an extra shot of regular before bed. I would get up at 3 A.M. and check my blood sugar. I had frequent episodes of low blood sugar during the night, but when we cut back my insulin, I had days upon end of waking up with sugars over 200. Many days I felt like a zombie, going through life in a slow, blurry daze, and I wanted to give up. I had gone from taking two shots a day and testing once or twice a day to taking five or more insulin shots a day and testing every few hours . . . and still my hemoglobin A1cs averaged around 8.5, well outside the normal range. I had embraced my diabetes, wanted to work with it and achieve healthy control, yet I was at the end of my rope, at a complete loss about what to do.

I had recently moved to Philadelphia to pursue graduate school and met a new endocrinologist, Ned Weiss. At our first meeting, Dr. Weiss and I talked about my diabetes, its effects on my quality of life, and my future plans. He suggested insulin pump therapy as the best alternative for me. He knew it would help me improve my diabetes control . . . and so improve my whole life. But I would not consider this option. I refused. The little I knew about insulin pumps (which was next to nothing) freaked me out. I was not about to attach some mechanical device to my body. That was all I needed! No thanks. I'd rather suffer and struggle through.

A few months went by. I was trying to keep up the busy pace of working and going to graduate school full-time. Finally, I became so frustrated with my diabetes control, I began to consider the pump. I decided that if I was going to make this kind of major decision about my life, I needed information. I read the brochures the pump companies produced; I studied John Walsh's *Pumping Insulin*. But while the brochures helped me learn about the basics of each particular pump and John Walsh's book helped me to understand the basics of how pump therapy worked, I wanted to know more. How would this (what felt monumental) choice affect my *whole* life—my sense of self, my body image, my relationships with others, my depression?

I embarked on a quest for knowledge and information to help me make the most informed decision about whether the pump was right for me. I learned that a major part of the process would be facing and breaking through my self-created fears and obstacles that were keeping me from choosing pump therapy. In the chapters ahead, I will share my process, and the stories of many other people with diabetes who've chosen insulin pump therapy, with you.

Choosing pump therapy has been one of the greatest choices I've ever made in my life. I have been pumping now for three and a half years . . . and I feel fantastic! I am a healthy, active, nondepressed person. My A1cs have stayed in the normal range, and I feel better than I have in my entire life. I am living my dreams in my personal and professional life, and feel optimistic about my future.

I know for sure that I would not be in the same shape if it weren't for my decision to try pump therapy. I have written this book in the hope that the stories and experiences of those who have chosen pump therapy will inspire you or your loved ones with diabetes to seriously consider this life-altering option for optimal diabetes control.

This is a book for the *whole* person with diabetes—examining the emotional, social, and spiritual as well as physiological dimensions of choosing to live with an insulin pump. Divided into five sections, *Insulin Pump Therapy Demystified* will guide you through the issues affecting the decision to choose pump therapy; explain (from the point of view of over seventy-five pump users) what it's *really* like to live with the pump; discuss what you need to do to prepare for successful pump therapy; delve into issues of maintenance for ongoing pump therapy success; and will also provide a specialized guide for insulin pump therapy for specific life situations—kids, teens, pregnant women, and senior citizens.

For my book, I spoke with countless diabetes educators, researchers, and experts, whose wisdom is invaluable. However, the bulk of the "expertise" comes from people just like you, whose own sharing of their experience adjusting to pump therapy can make your transition that much easier. Because insulin pump therapy is still a relatively new field, and because there have been comparatively few clinical trials on it (less than twenty worldwide, compared to thousands of studies on heart disease), pump therapy is a truly experiential process that requires the patient to take command of his or her diabetes care.

The good news is that all the clinical trials conducted so far have proven that insulin pump therapy, when practiced by motivated and educated pump users, leads to better control than multiple injection therapy. At the June 2002 annual meeting of the American Diabetes Association, three studies presented demonstrate that pump therapy is the most effective way to maintain tight blood sugar control, and can result in fewer diabetes-related complications. But pump therapy is not a cure for diabetes; the pump is not a magical device that you attach to and are able to leave your blood sugars worries behind. No, pump therapy—especially during your initial stage of adjustment— demands that you keep good records, accumulate data about how specific foods and activities affect your insulin requirements, and work closely with a physician or educator to find the correct amount of basal insulin that works for you. With pump therapy, the patient must be ready to go through a period of trial and error that can bring with it an initial feeling of frustration and doubt. But the thrill of pump therapy—despite this sometimes challenging stage—is that you, the pump user, will be in the driver's seat, in charge of your diabetes in a way that is simply not possible with any other insulin therapy.

Proper education about both the mechanics of the pump and the physiology of how pump therapy works in your body is essential before you get started. Especially if you have lived with diabetes for a long time and know intuitively how to draw up an injection and how long-acting insulin interacts in your body, it is important to bear in mind that you will be learning a whole new way to work with your diabetes. My Buddhist friends would say that this relearning requires a "beginner's mind"; that is, you have to let go of your comfort and expertise with the old system and get ready to try something that may feel very different and new.

It is critical that you find a health care provider who is experienced with pump therapy (I will discuss how to do so later in the book). Unfortunately, millions of people worldwide with diabetes are still taking injections because their physicians are not up-to-date with the latest research on the pump. In other words, imagine that someone comes to you and asks what the best device is on the market for watching movies in your home. Would you suggest they buy a Betamax player? Of course not—it's a dinosaur. Yet, while the pump is clearly the DVD player of diabetes treatment, many health care providers still prescribe the old regime.

The decision to choose pump therapy may feel overwhelming right now—and you are not alone in that feeling. My hope is that this book will address any fears and concerns, and will provide you with the direction to find the resources that you need to make a happy, healthy transition to pump therapy.

Best of luck! And happy pumping!

PART ONE

To Pump or Not To Pump?

IN THIS OPENING section we'll explore exactly what an insulin pump is, and why you may want to choose one for the management of your diabetes. In addition to considering some basic information about the pump, I will outline the three qualities necessary to make a successful transition to pump therapy: knowledge, support, and commitment.

ONE

What Is an Insulin Pump and Why Would I Want One?

IF YOU OR someone you love has diabetes and you've never seen an insulin pump up close, you're not alone. It is estimated that of the 17 million people worldwide with diabetes, 3.7 million of them must rely on daily insulin shots. Yet, only 10 to 12 percent of people with diabetes who must rely on insulin currently treat their condition with pump therapy (though these numbers prove to be growing).

First introduced with somewhat crude technology in the late 1970s, the pump was designed by scientists and physicians in an effort to mimic the functions of a healthy pancreas. The first insulin pumps were actually adapted from similar pumps that were used to deliver constant medicine to treat cancer patients undergoing chemotherapy. The very first pump developed was approximately the size of a backpack, and after modification a few years later was still the size of a large lunch box. Unfortunately, while the "theory" of pump therapy was sound, the initial practice of it was sometimes shaky. The technology to create a safe mechanical system was not yet in place; consequently, early pump users faced such challenges as not having adequate alarms to let them know when the pump was experiencing a technical malfunction.

From a lifestyle perspective, the pump required such unusual commitments as plugging it in every night and so not being able to move around while sleeping. Yet, many early pump users (some interviewed for this book) stuck with the system despite its flaws; they still achieved better blood sugar control on those pumps than they did with injection therapy. Fortunately, times have changed and today's pumps are small, sleek, and safe, and really do allow the user to "think like a pancreas" as the initial pump creators had envisioned. That is, just like a pancreas, an insulin pump releases small, continuous amounts of insulin into the bloodstream. In pump terminology, this is known as basal insulin. And just as a pancreas produces insulin quickly to counteract carbohydrate intake, an insulin pump allows its wearer to dial in additional insulin to cover the amount of carbohydrates ingested. This insulin is known as a bolus of insulin. The combination of correct basal insulin rates with additional bolusing allows the person with diabetes to achieve the closest thing possible to a functioning pancreas. With over thirty years of technology behind them, insulin pumps are now beeper-sized devices containing tiny computers, run on batteries. They are extremely safe, comfortable, and easy to wear.

Insulin is delivered through a thin tube that is connected both to the pump and to the person wearing the pump, through a needle or catheter, placed under the skin. Most pump users connect at the abdomen, although others use thighs, hips, upper buttocks, or even arms. The tube can be easily detached for some activities, such as showering, that are easier to do without the pump on. Insulin pumps allow their users to continue any physical activity they're involved in— they don't inhibit sports, recreation, work, or sex. In fact, because the pump user is able to lower the basal insulin rate during exercise or other activities that normally lower blood sugar, he or she will generally experience fewer hypoglycemic episodes.

As noted in the introduction, three recent clinical studies presented at the 2002 annual meeting of the American Diabetes Association indicate that "continuous subcutaneous insulin infusion with the assistance of a pump appears to be superior to multiple injections regarding metabolic control and clinical outcomes." That is, pump therapy allows the person with diabetes to achieve better blood glucose control than multiple injection therapy.

So—why aren't the other 88 to 90 percent of people with diabetes who take insulin shots rushing out to join those of us already on pump therapy? Certainly, any major change in diabetes treatment takes time to implement, and many participants are involved in making that change occur: physicians, educators, insurance companies, manufacturers, and most important, the patients themselves. As anyone living with diabetes knows, we must all act as our own advocates for getting the best health care possible, and very often it is the patient who must insist on making the switch to pump therapy. This chapter outlines reasons you may want to consider making the pump therapy change.

Yes, studies indicate that pump therapy improves blood sugar control. But I'm managing my diabetes okay. My control may not be perfect, but it's good enough. I'm comfortable with my routine of taking multiple injections. Why should I switch to pump therapy?

The answers to the above question are as diverse as the lives of any community of people living with diabetes. There is no "one reason" to make the change. The following profiles describe a sampling of real people living with diabetes and their struggles that led them to leave the comfort of their previous care behind in order to choose pump therapy.

CARYS PRICE grew up in Great Britain and now lives in the United States. In 1990, in her early thirties, she was a skinny, active person—who was diagnosed with diabetes. Initially, her doctor struggled to diagnose her as type 1 or type 2, but eventually started her on multiple injection insulin therapy. Long-acting insulin did not agree with her demanding job as a physical therapist, and by noon on most days she would find herself sweating, and "not feeling quite right" as low blood sugar came on.

YERACHMIEL ALTMAN, age forty-two, was diagnosed with diabetes at age two. He remembers his parents boiling his insulin needles, and how it felt not to be able to eat sweets like other kids. When he was twenty years old, he woke up one day with his vision greatly reduced. There were no laser treatments at that time to help his macular eye condition; he could only hope that it wouldn't get worse.

KIM SEELEY, an active thirty-three-year-old, became diabetic at age thirteen. In recent years, on multiple injection therapy, her A1cs ranged from 8 to 12. Even more frustrating than that was the regimented lifestyle that her diabetes demanded; Kim found it impossible to stick to a routine and wanted to be able to sleep late when she felt like it and eat out with friends.

DOREEN IS A SINGLE MOTHER WITH TWO TEENAGERS WITH DIABETES: JOE, FOURTEEN AND JESSICA, SIXTEEN. Joe also has cerebral palsy and Doreen struggled to help him to achieve good blood sugar control. Jessica's problems with long-acting insulin were worse though: She often had seizures from hypoglycemia and Doreen was willing to find any solution to this daunting challenge.

MORT WALDBAUM is seventy-five years old and has struggled with type 1 diabetes since his diagnosis forty-two years ago. He's gone through heart bypass surgery and has overcome alcoholism. But his diabetes had remained extremely brittle through it all, often causing Mort to pass out from hypoglycemia. In addition to those severe low blood sugar episodes, Mort's sugar would swing high so often that he couldn't get an A1c reading in the normal range.

Do any of these stories sound like yours? Do your struggles in living with diabetes resonate here? Each of the above individuals came to pump therapy out of a different need, yet each of them, as you will discover, improved his or her lifestyle and diabetes control by making the switch. Your reasons for considering and researching pump therapy are unique to you; yet many of us come to pump therapy because of the same frustrations with conventional multiple injection therapy.

TOP TEN

Reasons for Making the Change to Pump Therapy

1. Poor glucose control (high A1c values)

2. Frequent and/or nightly hypoglycemia

3. Desire for a flexible lifestyle (sleeping late, skipping meals, etc.)

4. Convenience—ease of taking insulin with the pressing of a button

5. Struggles with "dawn phenomenon" (rise in blood sugar during the early morning hours)

6. Variable nature of your work schedule (overnight shifts, air travel, food restrictions, etc.)

7. Desire for precise dosing (ability to take less than a half unit of insulin as needed)

8. Planned or existing pregnancy

9. Fluctuations in blood sugar control during monthly menstrual cycle

10. Better weight management and control with exercise

TWO

Seeking Knowledge

THE DECISION TO go on the insulin pump can be one of the most significant decisions you will make in your life. It is not an easy decision for many people and deserves serious time and attention. It is a decision that can dramatically change your life for the better, as it has done for me and the other people profiled in this book. The insulin pump can give you a sense of control over your diabetes that is not possible with shots or medication. The insulin pump gives you the power to work with your body in a constant, ongoing relationship. Still, many people with diabetes are reluctant to start pump therapy for one reason or another. The essential question for any person considering this therapy boils down to this: Are you ready and willing to take the challenge of going on the pump? The next few chapters will introduce you to the three important things you need to acquire before taking the pump challenge: knowledge, support, and commitment. Let's begin with knowledge.

I'm interested in exploring insulin pump therapy but need a lot more information before I determine if this is the right

way to go for me. Where can I turn to find out what I really need to know about living with the pump?

In all things we face in life, knowledge is power. Knowledge helps you make informed decisions; knowledge allows you to think critically and objectively. In the case of pump therapy, knowledge is the key to dispelling your myths and fears and giving you a sense of perspective. If you are thinking about pump therapy as an option to control your diabetes, start asking questions! As a teacher, I know the old adage is true: There are no stupid questions, no bad questions. Pump therapy is a relatively new development and many of us haven't met anyone on the pump. You are not alone in your curiosity about how the pump operates, how it will impact your diabetes, and how it will affect you as a *whole* person. It is critical to remember that you are not just your diabetes—you are a person with a complex life, full of relationships, challenges, and dreams. Pump therapy will impact every facet of your life—physically, emotionally, financially, and spiritually.

So, you begin forming questions about the insulin pump. Whom can you turn to for answers? A great starting point, of course, is with your endocrinologist. Both Yerachmiel Altman and Ernie Demba, another veteran of the early model insulin pump, were fortunate to have doctors involved in the research going on at the time who brought them information about pump use. But today many endocrinologists have some level of knowledge and experience in working with pump therapy, so your job is to find a physician with a high level of pump comfort. Mort Waldbaum remembers making the switch to such a doctor. "I had been going to the same doctor for years, and he really wasn't doing anything to help me. My A1cs were high and he would say, 'You're doing as good as can be expected.' So I decided to find a new doctor, and once I did, he suggested I get on a pump," Mort recalls.

Liessa Demba, Ernie Demba's daughter and herself a diabetic since age three, had had bad reactions to NPH (long-acting insulin) and problems with insulin absorption. Her endocrinologist prescribed Lantus insulin, which unfortunately made Liessa's blood sugar control much worse, giving her daily swings from 40 to 400. Liessa was very familiar with pump therapy, as she grew up with a father who had been on and off the pump for twenty years, and was now doing remarkably well on pump therapy. Still, Liessa's current doctor was reluctant to try her on a pump. So, Liessa made it her determination to find a doctor who would respect her wishes. "I did some research on endocrinologists in the area, chose one I thought would be best, and went into the office saying, 'I want a pump,'" Liessa explains.

If your doctor has not suggested pump therapy or is not familiar with pump therapy, you, too, may want to look for a new doctor. The most cutting-edge, well-informed endocrinologists will have taken the time to learn about the pump and are experienced in starting patients in pump therapy. A great endocrinologist will help educate and guide you through the process of getting started with the pump. If your doctor has not talked with you about the pump, feel free to ask him or her to recommend a colleague who is knowledgeable about the pump. A good doctor is secure enough to refer you to the specialist you need. If you have trouble finding a well-informed endocrinologist in your area, contact your local American Diabetes Association or Juvenile Diabetes Research Foundation, who can point you in the right direction. Also, for pumpers living in the United States, an Internet Web site, created and maintained by pump users, offers a state-by-state guide to endocrinologists whom they've used and respected. You can access this Web site at www.insulin-pumpers.org/pumpdocs.cgi.

If you live in a rural area or small town with limited medical treatment options, don't despair. It may mean that finding a health care team who can set you up on the pump will require some travel. When I was first diagnosed at age ten and was growing up in central Pennsylvania, there was no local pediatric endocrinologist in our area. My parents would pack me—and my siblings—into our station wagon and off we'd go for a two-hour ride to Children's Hospital in Pittsburgh. Although it was a bit inconvenient—and we'd generally wait two to three hours before my appointment was even called—I am grateful that my parents had the vision to find me the best health care out there. If you want to start pump therapy, look until you find the right health care team who can support your decision. The traveling will be well worth your time and expense.

Your doctor may also recommend you consulting with a diabetes educator. Certified diabetes educators are sometimes better informed about the day-to-day operations of the insulin pump than physicians. Diabetes educators are trained to help you work with your diabetes and can give you the facts you need to know about going on the pump. Again, your local ADA or JDRF can help you find the people you need to insure your successful transition to pump life. Also, you can go to the American Association of Diabetes Educators' Web site to find an index of educators closest to you: www.aadenet.org.

Sonia Seifert, a Chilean-born sixty-five-year-old woman, had struggled with diabetes for forty years. By working with diabetes educator Gary Scheiner (himself a type 1 diabetic on pump therapy), Sonia gained the necessary skills to use a pump successfully. "I am not exactly computer comfortable," she says. "Gary was like my panic button—I could call him with all my questions."

While doctors and educators are important resources, it is incumbent on the patient himself to become a real master of the basics of pump therapy. Not only is this learning gratifying, but it also gives one a sense of real ownership about making the pump choice. It is ultimately your body, your health that is at stake . . . not the doctor's. Look at your decision about choosing pump therapy as a great research project, as an opportunity for investigation. Think about the time you put into researching any major decision, like buying a new car, making a career change, or choosing a school for your children. Isn't your health at least equally important as these valuable things?

I've talked with my doctor about pump therapy and she's ready to help me try it out. But I have questions that I'm not exactly comfortable asking her—I mean, she doesn't wear the thing. Where can I go to find answers to my "real" questions?

If you are reading this book, you are already well onto your path of exploration. You will find out more about the real experiences of real people with diabetes, just like you.

But don't stop here—keep reading, keep asking, and keep talking!

The Internet has done so much to revolutionize diabetes education; with the click of a mouse, you can read about the latest research. A list of great Web sites that can help you learn more about pump therapy appears at the end of this chapter.

Some sites I recommend checking out include www.insulin-pumpers.org, which is run by a group of folks who pump insulin, and www.insulin-pumpers-r-us, another pumper-created Web site.

Through the Internet, you can also communicate directly with people who are using the pump. There is a listserv called "Insulin Pumpers Digest" that posts daily questions and responses from pump users around the world. You can subscribe to it and read firsthand about what pump users are talking about: IP@insulin-pumpers.org.

While on the Web, you can also connect to the sites of the major pump manufacturers: Animas, www.animas.com; Sooil (also known as DANA in the United States), www.sooil.com; Disetronic, www.disetronic-usa.com; and Medtronic MiniMed, www.min-imed.com. These sites contain lots of information about each manufacturer's specific pumps and what their companies have to offer you. It is recommended that you make contact with each company to find out which one makes the best product for you. Remember, pump manufacturers have a limited clientele—they should be fighting to get your business. Don't hesitate to call each company and speak with a customer service representative; connecting with a company that you trust is a key factor in making your decision.

It seems like a lot of the "real information" about pump therapy is found on the Web and I'm just not a computer person. How can I find pump users to connect with?

If you don't have Internet access, don't despair. Much as I love my e-mail, nothing beats talking to a real live person anyway! Ask your doctor or educator for names and numbers of their patients who are pump users. Most pump users I've met are more than happy to share their experiences with the pump. Ask for people who have had positive and negative experiences (yes, some people do have trouble adjusting). Remember, the more information you gather, the more prepared you will be to start your own pump therapy. When I was talking to a variety of pumpers before making my decision, I spoke with a woman who my doctor outright told me had had a miserable first year on the pump. When I spoke with her, she told me bluntly about her trials and tribulations. A water aerobics instructor, she needed flexibility in her life and was hoping the pump would provide her with that. She freely admitted that she, having been on multiple injections for years, was not ready for a new routine. Her resistance to change made the first few months of her pump using really rough. When I spoke with her, she had been on the pump nearly two years and was now thrilled with her new therapy. She suggested I really make sure I was ready for a change. I learned a lot from our conversation and thought long and hard about whether I was open or resistant to a new routine. Ultimately, I decided that a change for the betterment of my health would be worth losing the security I had from caring for my diabetes in the same way for over seventeen years!

Speak to as many different pump users as possible; each one will share his or her unique perspective. Look around you; most likely, someone in your life knows someone else who is on the pump. In my case, I was talking about my decision to go on the pump at graduate school one day. From just casually mentioning it, I discovered that a fellow student had an aunt who was on the pump. She gave me her aunt's phone number and I was most grateful to talk with her.

Kathy Kochan, a fifty-three-year-old author of cookbooks for people with diabetes, first heard about pump therapy by getting into a conversation with the woman who was taking her over-the-phone order for diabetes supplies. "I talk to everyone," Kathy says, "and this time I found out that this lady had two children with diabetes who were on the pump. Besides taking my order, she talked to me for a long time all about the pump, and that encouraged me."

Put it out there that you're thinking about going on the pump; someone in your workplace, school, church or synagogue, or other community will know someone who's on the pump already, with whom you can speak. Pump therapy is definitely spreading!

There's one more fantastic place to learn about pump therapy from the experts (yes, the experts are the pump users!): That place is an insulin pump support group. Many communities offer monthly groups where pump users come together, face-to-face, to learn about the latest research and to talk about their pumping. Check with your doctor, ADA, or JDRF chapter to find a support group near you. Kathy Kochan acknowledges how much her pump support group helped her make the transition to pump therapy. "I don't know what I'd do without them," she says. "Even though I've been on the pump for five years, I am still learning. I always learn from them."

A pump support group will welcome you with open arms and appreciate the decision-making process you're going through. Support is crucial to your success as a pumper . . . which is why the next chapter is dedicated just to that!

TEN PLACES

1. A great endocrinologist (Look at the list at www. insulin-pumpers.org/pumpdocs.cgi.)

2. A certified diabetes educator (Check out www.aadenet.org.)

3. The American Diabetes Association and Juvenile Diabetes Research Foundation

4. Internet sites listed on the following page

5. Insulin pumpers listserv: Ip@insulin-pumpers.org

6. The major pump manufacturers: Animas, Disetronic, Medtronic MiniMed, and Sooil

7. An informational seminar at your local hospital

8. From other people on pump therapy (Ask and you shall find them!)

9. An insulin pump support group near you

10. Diabetes magazines such as *Forecast* and *Monitor*

WEB SITE LINKS RELATED TO DIABETES AND PUMPING INSULIN

www.animascorp.com: Official Web site of Animas company

www.aadenet.org: American Association of Diabetes Educators; includes a "find an educator near you" feature

www.childrenwithdiabetes.com: Helpful site for parents of children with diabetes

www.danapumps.com: The American division of the Korean pump manufacturer Sooil

www.disetronic-usa.com: Official Web site of Disetronic, USA

www.diabetes.org: American Diabetes Association Web site

www.diabetesorg.com: Includes links to many diabetes-related sites

www.diabetes-exercise.org: Home page for the Diabetes, Exercise and Sports Association

www.diabetesnet.com/ishop: Online bookstore carrying diabetes-related titles

www.glycemicindex.com: The comprehensive and authoritative guide to the glycemic index, from the University of Sydney

www.idf.org/home: Home page for the International Diabetes Federation, providing information on diabetes from a global perspective

www.insulin-pumpers.org: Web site run by pump users; includes link to a pumpers' listserv

www.insulin-pumpers.org.uk: Organization of insulin pump users from the United Kingdom; includes information of funding the pump in the U.K.

www.insulin-pumpers-r-us.com: Pump-user-created Web site, full of basic pump information and live chat rooms.

www.jdrf.org: Juvenile Diabetes Research Foundation Web site

www.minimed.com: Official Web site of Medtronic MiniMed

www.ndep.nih.gov: From the National Institutes of Health, health education about diabetes

www.pumpwearinc.com: Full line of insulin pump accessories for children and adults

www.sooil.com: Official Web site of the Korea-based insulin pump manufacturer

www.63.193.241.211/gwen/pumpoz/index.html: Organization of insulin pump users from Australia

THREE

Finding Support

ANY CHANGE IN our lives—from the disruption of our day-to-day routines to major losses and shifts—causes stress. Even good changes—like new relationships, the birth of a child, finding your dream job—can cause waves of anxiety. Preparing yourself for a change can greatly help to reduce stress. Think back to a time in your life when a big change occurred—what support did you find to help you get through it?

Choosing pump therapy will bring many changes into your life. If you have had diabetes for a number of years, like me, you may not even be able to comprehend what life would be like without giving yourself daily shots! Even if your control is not where you want it to be with your current routine, at least you know how to give injections or take medicine; you know what results to anticipate. Pump therapy is a different approach to working with diabetes; small amounts of insulin will be delivered to you constantly, night and day. You will determine how much insulin to bolus for your meals, how much to reduce your basal rate before exercising. This new system requires that you be open-minded, patient, and ready to learn. It requires that you are gentle with your body while you're learning; it demands that you put your health into a priority position in your life.

Fortunately, you don't need to go through this learning process and adjustment by yourself. Sue Depinto, a sixty-five-year-old woman from Iowa, had battled diabetes for thirty-six years before going on pump therapy. Sue didn't know anyone on the pump but knew she would need the support of others going through the same thing, so she started her own support group. "We meet monthly, and people come from as far as an hour and a half away," she explains. "And we e-mail each other in between. We need that contact to get through."

I'm feeling a bit anxious about giving up multiple injection therapy; I mean, at least I know what the problems are with long-acting insulin and how to deal with them. Switching to pump therapy feels like a huge change and I have plenty of other things going on in my life right now. I don't want to burden my family with all of my doubts. . . .

Support can come in a variety of forms. You can find people around you who will listen and help assuage your fears, people who will be there when you need to vent frustrations. You may find support from your doctor or educator. Or, like Sue, you can find pump users who have gone through exactly what you're going through now who will be willing to be there for you, anytime, when you have questions or just need to talk. Find that support now as you begin your exploration of life with the pump.

The people in your life who normally give you support will be happy to help you with this process. Don't underestimate the importance of sharing your fears, anxiety, or concern with friends and loved ones. People who don't have diabetes can't mind-read; they may not understand what an important decision this choice is for you. When I was thinking about going on the pump, some of my friends didn't realize what a big deal this was for me. Through talking to them, I found a couple of close friends who were happy to listen to me and support me as I came closer to using the pump. It was critical that I communicated what I was going through to them; when I reached out, they came forward to listen, no matter what.

Similarly, Sonia Seifert found that finding the right emotional support was a critical piece in choosing pump therapy. Sonia recalls being a young woman in Chile, feeling the need to keep her diabetes to herself. "In those days," she says, "you hid your health problems. I didn't even tell my husband about my diabetes until just before we were married." But when Sonia, then a widow with one grown son, made the choice to go on pump therapy, she found herself really needing some emotional support. "It is amazing, how I can talk to friends of mine . . . who aren't diabetic, they are close friends, and they listen to me when I'm frustrated with one thing or another. That is enough to keep me going," she describes.

TEEN TIPS

Finding Someone Who Understands

FOR TEENAGERS living with diabetes, finding support can be a critical aspect of their health care. During the teen years, young men and women begin to break away from their parents and struggle to fit in with their peers, sometimes making choices that put their health at risk in order to gain social acceptance. Feeling isolated and alienated is not uncommon for many teens, and can be exacerbated for a teenager coping with diabetes on top of other developmental challenges.

If your teenager is considering pump therapy, finding another teen who is already on the pump, with whom your teen can talk, can be the necessary step to making pump therapy work for him or her. Ask your doctor or educator for phone numbers or e-mail addresses of teens to contact. Your teen may resist reaching out, and may resent your interference, but you can at least provide the contact information, then back off.

Sometimes finding an adult besides a parent, such as a teacher, family friend, or minister who is on the pump, with whom your teen can talk, also works well. While it is developmentally appropriate for a teen to act like "they don't need anybody," it is often during these difficult years that we need someone to listen—more than ever.

I'm really excited about making the switch to pump therapy. So why is everyone around me so jumpy when I talk about it? From my wife to my coworkers, it seems like going on the pump really freaks people out.

Of course, not all people in our lives are great sources of support. I found that there were people in my life who projected their own anxieties onto me. "Are you sure you can handle the pump?" "What if something goes wrong?" "How can you deal with having something attached to your body?" These questions came from their own insecurities; they didn't know if they could handle something like the pump. They were worried about how they would handle something going wrong. They couldn't imagine their own body with a pump. I had to step back and realize that their fears had nothing to do with my own self-knowledge and confidence. People are constantly projecting their fears onto us, not just about diabetes, but about everything! If people respond to you negatively when you talk about going on the pump, listen carefully. Is their concern coming out of fear? You don't need to take on anyone else's insecurity; find friends and loved ones who can offer you positive energy.

Kathy Kochan went through a similar experience when she was making her choice. "Some people in my family said, 'Why are you doing this?' They thought I was too vain to be able to wear this thing on my body. But I had decided that I wanted better blood sugar control, and nothing else mattered. I just had to ignore them," she recalls.

Of course diabetes affects family dynamics, and when you, as the person with diabetes, make a major decision about your health care, it does affect everyone else. Family members may not understand how much this choice, while initially time-consuming, can actually benefit your long-term health goals and help make you a more active, independent person. Including those people closest to you, whether friends or family members, in your decision-making process can give them the knowledge they need to in turn be able to support you.

Finally, if you don't have people in your life who can give you the support you need, it's a good time to reassess. What activities are you involved in that attract positive people? It may be time to explore joining a church or synagogue; many houses of worship offer healing services and other support groups for people in their congregations who are dealing with chronic illness. It may be time to start volunteering; giving to those less fortunate always brings back so many gifts in return. Wherever you turn, remember that you deserve support and love always . . . and you will find the support and love you need to help you decide if an insulin pump is right for you.

Just thinking about my diabetes makes me feel depressed. If I go on the pump, it seems like I'm going to have to think about coping with diabetes even more than before . . . and I just don't know if I can handle that.

About six months before I made my decision to choose pump therapy, I started going to psychotherapy. I had been in therapy before and had battled with bouts of depression on and off for the last ten years. In the past, I had never focused on my diabetes as an issue to work on in therapy; I had never connected it to my depression. This time, I knew that having diabetes was really on my mind and so I sought out a therapist who could work with me on clarifying what emotional issues I had surrounding my illness. My therapist, Pam Ladds, is a registered nurse in addition to being a social worker. She also has family members with diabetes. Many of her cousins have diabetes and her late grandmother had diabetes, so Pam knew about this illness from real life, not just books. She helped me see that diabetes itself was not the problem, but, rather, my attitude around it was what was causing me grief. I was harboring feelings that somehow I was "damaged goods" because of my illness; I was not as perfect as I should be. I started thinking about the unhealthy way our culture treats illness and people with illness; how scared we are of our bodies, our mortality, the very fragility of life. In my therapy, I started realizing how much power I have in making my life what I dream it to be—one of good health, good relationships . . . a life of gratitude and growth. As I gained confidence about taking care of myself, my hidden feelings of self-pity and hopelessness began to dissipate. Diabetes is an enormous responsibility. It is natural to get sick of it, to resent it, to wish it would just go away. But the reality is, there isn't a cure right now, so we need to find the best way to live with it. For me and for so many others, going on the insulin pump has made diabetes so much more livable and controllable. I can't imagine going back to dealing with the unpredictability of long-acting insulin and the regiment of scheduled mealtimes.

I think of diabetes now as a gift rather than a burden; taking good care of myself helps me to realize that each day is sacred. I don't take life for granted and I am working hard to make my life last as long as possible. I couldn't have reached this philosophy without doing some serious emotional work in therapy and without finding friends and loved ones who supported me through the process of choosing pump therapy. As strange as it may sound, a chronic illness doesn't need to be a dreadful sentence. Each human being is given challenges and limitations; yet it seems to me that the beauty and dignity of the human condition is that we possess the power to overcome our adversities. I don't walk around jumping for joy that I have diabetes; yet in quiet moments, as I reflect on the journey of my life, I realize that I am a stronger, more compassionate, more loving human being because I have worked so hard, and continue to work, to create a healthy body, spirit, and mind. Chronic illness offers us the opportunity to assess what is truly important in life, and to reject the notion that a physical imperfection makes life any less worthwhile.

What support do you need in order to make your diabetes more livable? Is it pump therapy? Find the emotional support you need today to find out. Your life is worth it.

TEN REASONS

TO SEEK EMOTIONAL SUPPORT
IN CHOOSING PUMP THERAPY

1. Any change—even good changes—produces anxiety.

2. Learning new things, especially when you're giving up the "comfort" of your old ways of doing things, can be stressful.

3. While going through this new learning process, you may want someone who can listen to your frustrations.

4. You may feel isolated and want to talk to someone who can understand what you're going through, like a fellow pump user.

5. This change will affect family dynamics and can cause anxiety and fear in family members other than the person with diabetes.

6. Some people around you will make negative comments or react in an unsupportive way to this choice. Remember, it's *their* issue, not yours.

7. Issues about how you feel about living with diabetes may surface as you take on this new commitment.

8. It's healthy to take "emotional stock" of how you're doing with your diabetes.

9. Supportive people—especially those on-line buddies—can help you when that 3 A.M. panic (what in the world am I doing?) hits!

10. The more support you receive, the more you will be able to give to others—in all aspects of life—in return.

FOUR

Making the Commitment

NO MATTER HOW much knowledge you gather, nor how much support you receive, the success of your pump therapy ultimately lies with you. We all have times in which we work hard at our diabetes control, and other times in which we fall into a slump. Choosing to go on pump therapy is about making a commitment to tight control. As I've expressed earlier in this section, the pump puts more control into your hands than do shots or medication. I mean this quite literally; by pushing buttons to increase or decrease your basal rates and by deciding how much bolus to give, you are constantly active in your blood sugar control.

When I first heard about the pump, this factor really intimidated me. I had had so many experiences in which I had tried hard to achieve tight control and something always went wrong. How would I be able to handle using the pump, which would require so much work on my part? As I spoke to pump users, I heard a recurring theme time and again: Control, though requiring more constant monitoring and adjusting, is actually *easier* on the pump. "Easier" was something I could use! I realized that my blocks to tight control weren't my fault; my doctor and I just couldn't find the right dosage of insulin to deal with my dawn phenomenon. With the help of the pump, we could make easier adjustments that would allow me to fine-tune my diabetes care. When all else failed, I knew I was ready to make the commitment to the pump despite my fears. I knew my life was worth it.

I test my blood sugars before every meal and usually before I go to bed. I really hate pricking my fingers. Is that enough for good control with pump therapy?

"The bottom line with pump therapy," says Kim Seeley, "is that this thing is a machine. That's it—a machine. A lot of people go on the pump thinking they're getting a pancreas, but you're not. It's up to the pump user to take responsibility for good control."

What Kim points out could not be more true. To make pump therapy as successful as it can be requires more diligence in blood glucose monitoring. Because you don't have long-acting insulin in your system, it is critical to identify high blood sugars immediately and take the needed steps to break them down. In all honesty, I do test my blood sugars more now than I did before going on the pump (probably an average of eight to ten times a day). I do adjust my doses through the day to cover the activities I'm engaged in.

The candidates who are most likely to succeed with pump therapy are those people who want the tightest blood sugar control possible. Ernie Demba, who was diagnosed with type 1 diabetes at age fifteen, recalls his decision to try the first, experimental insulin pump. "I had two kids who were diabetic and I knew the pump was ultimately the best way to get good blood glucose control. I was willing to let them experiment on me so that the pump would be better for my kids. I wanted to stick around, for them . . . no matter," he says.

A Commitment for Mom and Dad

IF YOU are the parent of a child (or children) with diabetes, the willingness to commit to pump therapy falls on you as much as on your child. Especially for parents of young children, it is essential that you are willing to take on the challenge of "thinking like a pancreas"—even when that pancreas doesn't belong to you, and is actively engaged in school, sports, and social activities.

Don't despair—pump therapy can offer incredible benefits in flexibility for your family, and even more important, can offer better blood sugar control for your child. But these benefits come only if you can commit fully to the task of being the primary pump therapy decision-maker, until your child reaches a level of emotional and intellectual maturity at which time he or she can take on some of the tasks, such as testing blood sugars and determining boluses on his or her own.

Talk to other parents of young pumpers and find out what helped them to make the pump therapy commitment.

I'm willing to test my blood sugar more than I'm doing now. What other "commitments" do I need to make to be a successful pumper?

Pumping insulin requires a willingness to do frequent testing and ability to make decisions, along with your doctor's input, of course, based on that data. It requires a commitment to "checking in" on your machine—having insulin cartridges and new batteries always with you and ready to go. It means changing infusion sites regularly and cleaning your skin to avoid infection.

When I first started pumping, these "commitments" felt new and a bit daunting. But all of this fine-tuning is second nature to me now . . . it is not burdensome in any way. I feel so much better physically, my energy has increased, and I am reassured when my blood sugars can stay in the normal range. My commitment to pumping—once a struggle—is now like an established relationship. We still have our moments—as all "couples" do—and I know that's healthy—but we're ultimately together for the long haul.

All this having been said, bear this notion in mind. The pump is not permanently attached in any way. If it doesn't work for you, you won't be forced to stay on pump therapy. If you would rather, you can always go back to your previous care routine. Sonia Seifert actually decided to go off pump therapy the first time she tried it. She was already on the pump for two years, struggling a bit with the mechanics, until she finally decided that "this thing was not for me!" Sonia went back to multiple injection therapy but couldn't achieve as good blood sugar control as she had while on the pump. "The second time I tried the pump, it was my decision. The first time, it was really my doctor who wanted me to do it. But the second time, I made the commitment. That made all the difference in the world," she notes.

TEN COMMITMENTS

You Need to Make to Be a
Successful Insulin Pumper

1. Willingness to test blood sugar up to 8 to 10 times a day

2. Willingness to carry pump batteries, insulin cartridges, back-up insulin, and syringes with you at all times

3. Ability to master mechanics of the pump

4. Ability to analyze blood sugar data and make adjustments to basal rates as needed

5. Figure out carbohydrates of the food you're eating and how to bolus accurately for them

6. Remember to check on "mechanics" of the machine—are there large air bubbles in your tubing? Is your infusion site okay?

7. Work with health care team to make ongoing adjustments

8. Periodically review basal rates for correctness

9. Check ketones when blood sugars are high (over 250 mg/dL)

10. Test blood sugar (periodically) in the middle of the night

PART TWO:

What's It Really Like to Live with the Pump?

AS ANYONE LIVING with diabetes knows, health professionals are a great resource and source of help, but is you—and you alone—who knows what it *feels* like to live with the ups and downs of this disease. Communicating with other folks with diabetes can provide a sense of solidarity, although each of us experiences diabetes uniquely.

The same applies to the experience of life with the insulin pump. Our doctors and educators can teach us what we need to learn about how to manage pump therapy, but it is really from other pump users that we can learn what it *feels* like to be on a pump. And, of course, one pump user's experience may be totally different from another person's experience.

Nonetheless, in this section of the book, we will examine the real-life experience of pump users, coming to grips with some of those topics that are, well . . . a bit *uncomfortable* to talk about in the doctor's office, the topics that make us feel nervous or resistant when we think about choosing pump therapy.

"The only thing we have to fear is fear itself." Franklin D. Roosevelt's famous words proved to be absolutely true to me once I started pumping. It was really quite incredible just how many different fears my mind had concocted while I was considering going on the pump. While I'm generally a positive person, I reacted so strongly with fear to the idea of pump therapy because it felt like such an overwhelming challenge. I had to break down my fears one by one. I couldn't address some of them until I was actually on the pump. I realize that I am not alone in "imagining catastrophe"; many of us fantasize about the worst. Whenever I talk to people who are considering pump therapy, the conversation always turns to "I like the idea, but, well, what about—" And then they name their personal list of fears! Hopefully, the next seven chapters address whatever fear or lingering doubt may be eating away at you. This is the real thing—what it feels like to live with an insulin pump, from the experiences of those who are doing so.

FIVE

Body Image, Fashion, and Visibility

WHEN MY DOCTOR initially explained the pump to me, I just kept thinking, "Where does this thing *go*? What am I going to look like with this *thing* sticking out of me? I will be a total freak!" Of course at that time, I hadn't actually seen a pump and I didn't believe my doctor that it was as small as a beeper and pretty much looked like one. Yeah, right! A little beeper-thing is going to be able to deliver my insulin night and day? I don't think so!

When I finally saw a pump, my disbelief was shattered. It was small. It didn't look scary. Still, I thought, I like to wear skirts and dresses and bathing suits. . . . I'm not going to be able to find a way to wear this thing and still look good!

Well, the fear of being unattractive was shattered when Nicole Johnson was crowned Miss America in 1999. While I'm not someone who normally pays attention to beauty contests, I couldn't help but be inspired by Nicole. The insulin pump was getting national press coverage. She wore her pump in everything but the swimsuit contest, and she looked amazing! Heck, she was picked to be Miss

America! Like many other women, I saw Nicole as a role model: confident and strong, putting diabetes control as a top priority in her life.

I'm a real "clotheshorse," love dressing in tight-fitting styles. Where do I put this thing so that it doesn't totally ruin my fashion statement?

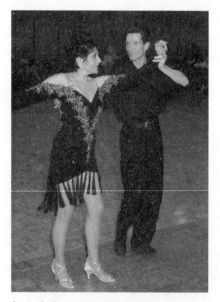

Sonia Seifert, pump user and ballroom dancer

Sonia Seifert also had initial doubts about wearing the insulin pump. "How am I going to live with this thing, as a woman?" she asked. Sonia spent some time experimenting to find the right clothing that made her look and feel good. "The pump is easy to clip on skirts or pants, but it's harder if you have something like a wedding to attend and want to wear a fancy dress. Where do you put it?" One solution Sonia has found is to wear a fancy blouse with a sash for more formal events, so that she can still clip her pump onto a skirt. Sonia, who is a national award-winning ballroom dancer, does disconnect from the pump during dance competitions when she wears very tight-fitting dresses. By monitoring her blood sugar closely and taking an insulin injection if necessary, Sonia is able to make that compromise and maintain good blood sugar control. "Give a woman a clothing challenge—and she'll find a way around it," sums up Kim Seeley's feelings about wearing her pump and still feeling attractive. Kim found that wearing tight pants with a looser blouse is an easy way to "hide" the pump. She still wears backless halter tops, keeping her pump in a special athletic pouch she wears on her upper thigh. For formal engagements, she's even had a seamstress sew a discreet pocket into a dress for her insulin pump.

Kathy Kochan originally feared that her vanity would get in the way of her decision to choose pump therapy, but once she made the move, she's had no regrets. "I gave away my A-line dresses, " she recalls, "but other than that, I've found a way to wear the pump with everything. A padded bra from Victoria's Secret works wonders."

Before I went on the pump, I ordered a few different "devices" to help me wear the pump without compromising my fashion ideals. I have a product called "the thigh thing" that consists of a little spandex garter with a pocket—my pump slides right in. I always wear it with dresses and skirts. It's kind of fun and sexy—knowing I have my garter on! When I got married in June 2001, I wore the thigh thing with my insulin pump under my wedding dress and no one saw a thing. Just a happy, healthy bride!

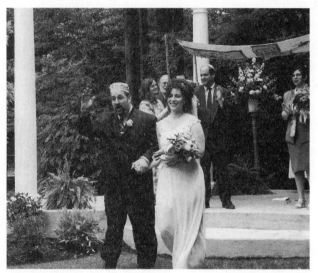

The author on her wedding day, June 24, 2001. Can you spot her pump?

Of course, one person's solutions is another's . . . shall we say . . . challenge? When Kathy Kochan tried to wear a "thigh thing," she nearly lost her garter and her pump as she was walking down the aisle in church one morning! "You've got to keep a sense of humor with this thing," Kathy says, still laughing. For many women with thinner thighs, this alternative is not the best. But again, between padded bras and special pockets, there are numerous ways to wear your pump with almost any fashion.

Another bride I spoke to, Judy Swenson, just did not want to have to worry about her insulin pump on her big day. "I'm usually a shorts and T-shirt person, so I don't give a thought to wearing my pump and how I look. Most people think it's a beeper anyway. But for my wedding, I wanted to look really beautiful . . . and the dress I found was strapless and pretty form-fitting. I didn't want to deal with people looking at my pump rather than at me," she explains. Judy's doctor helped her plan for her wedding day by having her practice taking off her pump for 5 to 6 hours (the time she'd actually be in her wedding dress) and taking injections of regular insulin during that time. "On my wedding day," Judy recalls, "I had my bridesmaid pull me aside and we checked my blood sugar every hour. I was too excited to eat, so my sugars stayed pretty steady. It was actually a relief to change out of the dress and reconnect to my pump later on."

As I wrote earlier, each pump user approaches the challenges of life with the pump differently. Still another bride, Cara Jennings, decided to incorporate her insulin pump case into the design of her wedding dress. Cara, a graphic artist and a very creative lady who made her own wedding ensemble, covered her pump case with the same fabric she used to make her two-piece dress. She clipped her pump onto her waistband, and wore it just as she would any other day. Making your pump case into a fashion accessory seems to be catching on, especially with the teenage and twenty-something set. With funky fabric, sequins, rhinestones, and stickers, pumpers are creating a new trend with their original cases. The Animas pump even comes with changeable stickers!

TEEN TIPS

What to Do About Prom Night

IT'S IMPORTANT for parents to remember that even if you can barely recall the feeling now, going to the prom may seem like the most important thing in the world to your teenager. Looking good—for both guys and gals—is essential.

Teenage boys have it pretty easy—tuck the pump in a tuxedo pocket, and off you go. Girls may find it more challenging to wear the dress of their dreams with a pump. Parents can help by taking daughters to a seamstress to have an original creation made, or asking the seamstress to add a discreet pocket to an existing dress.

If your daughter insists that she is *not* wearing her pump for prom night, don't fight her. Instead, make an appointment with your doctor or diabetes educator and figure out a safe strategy for her to switch to injections for the night.

And even if her prom date doesn't turn out to be Prince Charming, and if years from now you'll both laugh at the now out-of-date dress she just had to have, she will remember one thing: your love and support and the extra mile you went to make living with diabetes not so bad.

You'll find the way to wear your pump to best suit you—clipped on a belt, tucked away in a pocket, covered by a blazer or a sport coat. You will find the right way to wear your insulin pump and still look fabulous!

SUCCESS STORY

An Interview with Nicole Johnson, Miss America 1999

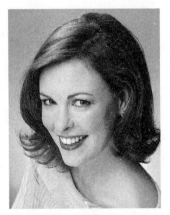

Miss America 1999, pump user and diabetes advocate Nicole Johnson

PUMP USER Nicole Johnson, who was chosen as Miss America 1999, has served as an inspiration for many people. She has been an outspoken advocate for diabetes education and fund-raising for diabetes research. As the first Miss America with diabetes (and on the insulin pump), Nicole has spoken openly and honestly about living with diabetes. Her personal story is chronicled in her book, *Living with Diabetes*.

I had the good fortune to connect with Nicole and ask her about her experience in choosing pump therapy.

GKM: How long have you had diabetes and when did you first learn about the insulin pump?

NJ: I've had diabetes for almost ten years now. I first saw an insulin pump at an expo meeting in Virginia in 1997 and was intrigued.

GKM: What influenced your decision to choose pump therapy?

NJ: I wanted better control over my diabetes. I wanted to improve my odds against complications and I wanted to lessen the number of hypoglycemic episodes I was having. Ultimately, a severe hypoglycemic event at the 1997 Miss Virginia Pageant led to my going on the pump.

GKM: How did your transition to the pump go? What was the hardest part of pump therapy to master?

NJ: My transition was rather smooth. I was used to the device in a matter of days. It was probably 2 to 3 weeks until I felt totally comfortable. The hardest part was inserting the cannula.

GKM: How has pump therapy changed your life? How did it affect your work as Miss America?

NJ: I couldn't have done my job of being Miss America without the pump. It gave me the flexibility and the freedom I needed to be successful. I was able to travel twenty thousand miles a month and stay in good control of my diabetes thanks to the pump. I really credit the device with saving my life and giving me my life's work.

GKM: How did you deal with fashion concerns and the pump during pageants?

NJ: I was able to wear the pump during the Miss Virginia and Miss America pageants. I wore the pump in many different places. For example, during the evening wear section of the pagaent, I had the pump on the inside of my thigh. Thigh control panty hose held it in place.

GKM: Do you have any fashion tips for day-to-day life with the pump?

NJ: I also wear the pump in my bra, under my arm, or clipped to boots during the winter (with the long tubing). Usually my pump is clipped to my waist. I almost always have the pump resting in the small of my back when I am working or wearing a business suit. I am not ashamed of the device and therefore don't put much effort into hiding it anymore. Everyone expects to see it on me.

GKM: What was the best part of sharing your Miss America platform?

NJ: I was sharing my heart—my platform was and still is me. It was liberating to be so honest about my diabetes. I loved seeing people come to terms with their own conditions through my terms. As people saw me talk openly about my struggles, it gave them a little freedom and nudging to do the same. That is what I am most thankful and grateful for. I hope that I helped people release and dispel the negative stigma that often accompanies a chronic disease like diabetes.

GKM: What advice would you give to people considering pump therapy?

NJ: DO IT! You will not be sorry. Intensive therapy is really the only way to successfully manage your diabetes and ward off the threat of complications. I think the pump is for anyone who is motivated to live a full and wonderful life in spite of their diabetes. It is for anyone who is willing and ready to beat the odds. It is for anyone who wants to live complication free! Until there is a cure, pump therapy is the answer—at least it is for me!

I don't think I'll mind wearing an insulin pump, but I don't like the idea of people noticing it and coming up to me all the time, asking me what it is. How do I deal with that?

I know that body image and fashion concerns about the pump may be more of an issue for women than men. In fact, none of the men I spoke to—from college-age students to older men like Mort Waldbaum, seemed to worry about their body image or having an insulin pump fashion emergency.

But the issue of visibility is something that concerns both men and women. When you have diabetes, you are generally able to "pass" for a person without a chronic condition; having diabetes doesn't make you look any different from anyone else. For people who prefer not to share their diabetes and regard it as a personal matter, choosing to wear a pump may seem to threaten their privacy.

First of all, if you don't want the pump to be visible to others, it doesn't have to be. As I discussed above, there are many ways to work with your clothing to make the pump work for you. Often times, I have the pump tucked away and people have no idea I'm wearing it, based on my appearance.

"The only time anyone's ever asked me about my pump is in the gym," Kim Seeley says. "And then they want to know if it's a heart monitor or some other high-tech fitness thing. In day-to-day life, no one's ever said a thing to me. People are too self-centered to notice." Indeed, most pump users are rarely asked about their pump; if they are, those asking often assume it's a new kind of beeper or cell phone and want to know where they can get one.

I relate to the concern of explaining the pump to people because I used to hate talking about my diabetes. I had enough trouble dealing with my diabetes, besides discussing it with the world. I found that when people talked about diabetes, it often involved "doom and gloom" stories—about a relative with complications or some other negative tale. I didn't want to hear it. But when I got the pump, I was so excited about feeling good, it didn't matter to me anymore if people knew about my diabetes. I wore my pump out on my belt when it was convenient, and if people asked me what it was, I happily explained it to them.

One of the nicest things that's happened as a result of wearing my pump is that I've been able to help and affect other people with diabetes. Some people who've noticed my pump and asked me about it have a friend, parent, spouse, or child with diabetes. I've been able to show them how easy the pump is to wear and use and to talk with them about the benefit of pump therapy. I've helped a few total strangers get started with their pumping, and this process is what initially inspired me to write this guide.

Liessa Demba, who's been on the insulin pump for almost a year, made a conscious decision to wear her pump out, on a belt or clipped to a pocket, so that she could see it. "It's just like wearing a watch to me, and I wanted to be able to see it easily to make adjustments," she explains. In her job as education director of a large religious school, Liessa is in contact with over three hundred children a week. "I wanted them to be able to see the pump, and ask me questions about it," she says. "They want to learn about diabetes."

Rather than being a negative thing that people see my pump, it has opened an ongoing dialogue and network. And when I am feeling private and don't want to share my pump with the world, I can wear it under my clothes and it is goes unnoticed.

Nonetheless, some pump users have encountered the occasional negative reaction when a stranger (or even friend or acquaintance) notices the pump. "How can you stand being attached to that thing?" they may ask. If that should happen to you, it is important to recognize that it is *their* insecurity that is coming up in the question. It may be that because you've always looked healthy, friends and loved ones may not think about your diabetes much and suddenly, your wearing the pump may become a physical reminder of your condition. If they are uncomfortable dealing with your diabetes, it may come out in an expression about the pump. The important thing for you to do is to be clear with them about why you've chosen pump therapy and how beneficial it is in your life. In most cases, this rational behavior will eclipse their negativity.

I'm not so worried about how I'll look wearing an insulin pump, and I don't care if people notice and ask me about it, but I worry about how it will feel. It seems so artificial to go around with this little computer thing connected to your skin. I don't know if I can handle that.

Again, everyone, men and women, children and teenagers, may be thinking about that lingering image of "having something attached" to their body. I can honestly assure you that within a few days, you will grow so used to wearing the pump that it won't feel strange at all. It really becomes just a part of your body. About a week after I got my pump, I was in the car, driving somewhere. Suddenly, I felt myself panic—oh, my goodness, I'm not wearing my pump! What did I do? Did I take it off somewhere? When I got to a stoplight, I looked down and of course it was still there, connected to the infusion site in my abdomen! I had just stopped being aware of it. It was part of me, just like an arm or a leg, working all the time to keep my life going but noticeable only when I focused on it.

Yerachmiel Altman remembers well the old days, over twenty years ago, when the insulin pump was a big, cumbersome thing . . . that you couldn't forget was attached to you. Every eighteen to twenty-four months, he would try a newer, more updated version of the pump, that was invariably smaller and more comfortable to wear. "When I think of where we've come," he reflects, "it's really so amazing. Today's pumps are light, sleek, and easy to wear. I wouldn't tell anyone to think twice about wearing one."

TEN WAYS
TO CONQUER BODY IMAGE/FASHION/ VISIBILITY CONCERNS

1. Before you start pumping, experiment with different styles of clothing that could work well with the pump.

2. Look on-line at pump accessory catalogues, such as www.pumpwearinc.com.

3. For women, visit a Victoria's Secret and figure out which bra style can help you discreetly tuck away your pump.

4. Find a seamstress or tailor who can work with you in creating pockets in your favorite dresses.

5. Make your pump clip case into a funky fashion accessory.

6. Find the insertion site that is most comfortable for you. While most people use the abdomen, others find inserting on the hip or thigh to be more comfortable.

7. If you have a special occasion like a prom or wedding coming up and you really don't want to wear your pump, talk with your doctor about switching to injections for a few hours.

8. Remember, it's your call whether you want to wear the pump out in a "visible" way or tuck it away, where no one will notice it, such as in a pocket or clipped to a bra. You can change how you wear your pump based on how you're feeling that day.

9. Prepare short responses to people's questions if you're uncomfortable talking with strangers about the pump. And if you want to be a "pump teacher," encourage others' questions when they want to know about the pump.

10. Examine your anxiety about people knowing about your diabetes. What's behind it? How can you feel less anxious about talking about it?

SIX

Sleeping with the Pump

DON'T KNOW why, but when I first heard about the pump, I kept thinking, "Well, what do you do with it at night?" The idea of *sleeping* with this thing attached to me seemed totally strange and impossible. It is a common concern; I repeatedly hear, "But you don't sleep with it, do you?" "Back in the old days," says veteran Ernie Demba, "it was quite a challenge to sleep with an insulin pump. Awful. The thing was so big, you couldn't change positions. But that's a concern of the past. I've never had trouble sleeping with my new pump."

In fact, sleeping can be more pleasurable than ever for the person living with diabetes. "I just love being able to sleep late!" exclaims Kim Seeley. "No more waking up early on those days you could sleep in because you must get that morning shot in." Amen!

I'm a very sensitive sleeper and can't imagine sleeping with the pump "in me." That's my only real doubt about trying the pump, but it's a big one.

I can empathize with this concern and understand its magnitude. I'm a pretty sensitive sleeper too. I toss and turn sometimes and I always change positions in my sleep. I was scared to death that I would tear the pump out of me during the night.

This has never happened, and it never will. The pump is secure and strong; people play football with it! A little tossing won't hurt a thing. My sleep has been sound all through my pump using . . . but I had to try sleeping with the pump to actually believe it.

But where do you put the pump while you sleep?

Again, check out all the insulin pump accessory lines and you'll find pajamas designed for both men and women with special pockets for the pump. Personally, I prefer buying cute pajamas—just so they have a top and bottom—to clip it onto at night.

David Cohen, a twenty-one-year-old college student, hasn't let the pump interfere with his preferred nighttime style: sleeping in the buff. "I just put the pump on the bed beside me, and it's fine. I guess I roll around a little, but the pump stays pretty much in the same place I put it when I went to bed. Sleeping nude is part of my lifestyle, and I couldn't see giving that up," Dave says proudly.

What about all of those beeping buttons and alarms? Doesn't the pump disrupt your sleep?

The insulin pump is equipped with alarms that will wake you if need be. If your batteries are low at 3 A.M., the pump will beep and keep beeping until you turn it off.

The alarms are loud enough that they should wake even the soundest of sleepers. (Unfortunately, that means that they can wake partners too!) Though it's a pain in the butt, an occasional alarm going off is much preferred to sleeping through a mechanical glitch. It's a pretty infrequent occurrence and rated at the bottom of the list of concerns among insulin pumpers that I spoke with.

"If my insulin cartridge is getting low," says Judy Swenson, "I change it *before* I go to bed. I learned that the hard way, by getting woken up at 4 A.M. with a cartridge-low warning. Even if I still have a little insulin left in the cartridge, it's worth it to change it at 11 P.M. rather than trying to be alert at those early hours."

Pumps and Sleepovers

SLEEPOVERS AND slumber parties are an important part of most kids' social lives. There's no reason that kids who pump can't join in the fun!

Parents just need to check in with the parents of your child's friend (who are, of course, responsible people or you wouldn't let your child sleep there to begin with!). Make sure that they understand that the pump *stays on your kid all night*. Next, make an action plan with them for blood sugar testing and bolusing. For example, many parents like to be called at snack time so they can quickly instruct their kids on how much to bolus, based on what the kid will be eating. And another quick check-in before breakfast can insure good blood sugar control into the next day.

What about that tubing stuff?
Doesn't it get twisted while you sleep?

Again, sleeping with the pump has rarely proved to be a problem for most pumpers.

Tubing can be neatly tucked into pajamas, and won't tangle at all. Tubing also comes in different lengths, so you can find the length that works best for you.

I had one more fear about sleeping with the pump. I have two cats, the loves of my life, who usually sleep with me. I was afraid that during the night they might chew the tubing or try to yank it out. Miraculously, they, who are curious about anything and everything, have never come near my pump! Cats are so brilliant—they must intuitively know to stay away. (Well, most cats anyway!) Still, if you have pets or any other thing that could potentially interfere with your nighttime safety, take precautions. Your health is worth it, and so are your dreams!

TEN WAYS

TO ENJOY GOOD SLEEP
WITH THE PUMP

1. Find several good pairs of pajamas or nightshirts that you can easily clip the pump onto. Also, check out on-line pump clothing sites for specially designed pump pajamas.

2. Keep some glucose tabs on a bedside table should you wake up with low blood sugar during the night.

3. Before you go to sleep, check your blood sugar (of course!) and check to make sure that your insulin cartridge or reservoir is full enough to get you through the night.

4. Keep batteries in a convenient place by your bed in case you need to make a quick change.

5. Placing a small lamp close by can help you read your pump screen quickly if an alarm does go off (or use your pump's back light if it has one).

6. Alert your sleep mate to the sounds of your pump alarm so that he or she can help to wake you up if an alarm goes off.

7. Shut your bedroom door if curious pets make any attempt to chew on or pull at your pump tubing.

8. If you tend to move around an unusual amount during the night and/or are a violent sleeper, talk to your diabetes educator about using extra adhesive tape to keep your infusion site in place.

9. Enjoy the pleasures of sleeping late! With proper basal rates set, insulin pump therapy means that you don't have to wake up early to take a morning insulin shot.

10. Periodically, you will need to wake up and check your blood sugar during the night to make sure that basal rates are set at the correct rate.

SEVEN

And Now, Ladies and Gentlemen . . . the Question You've All Been Waiting for: Sex and the Pump!

OKAY, OKAY. I was worried about how I'd look with the pump . . . I was worried about sleeping . . . but I was downright terrified that having the insulin pump might interfere with my sex life! I mean, where do you put this thing when you're doing it?

I was single when I was first considering pump therapy, and I was scared that future partners might be put off by the pump. Sure, I thought, if you're already with a partner who loves and accepts you . . . then what's to worry about? But I was young and active and the thought of the pump precluding my sex life was perhaps the strongest barrier to my considering it.

I am totally freaked out about a potential sex partner finding out about this "thing" attached to my body. What a turnoff. How do I deal with my pump in the bedroom?

Among pump users I spoke with, I discovered that both single people of all ages and circumstances, some in committed relationships for years, and married folks, felt some degree of anxiety about whether they would still be an attractive partner with the insulin pump. Dave Cohen remembers going on the pump just before his freshman year in college, and wondering whether girls would be put off by the pump. "I definitely knew the pump was the only way to go for college, because my schedule would be crazy and I wanted to eat whenever I felt like it. Still, I kept thinking, are girls going to be grossed out by this thing? Can you still have sex with a pump on?" Dave admits to thinking.

Dave's early concerns are echoed by many of people considering pump therapy. Sexuality is an important part of life and developing a healthy body image. For people living with diabetes, who may feel "different" from other so-called "healthy" people, sexuality is an opportunity not only to connect intimately with others but also to prove that our bodies are strong and capable and sensual. The idea that an insulin pump could threaten our sexual self-esteem seems like a tenuous trade-off for good blood sugar control.

Now that I'm older and wiser, I've learned from personal experience and from talking to other pumpers that despite those initial worries, the insulin pump will absolutely *not* interfere with your sex life! In fact, in most cases, it will actually *improve* it! I mean, doesn't it make sense that if you're feeling better physically, you'll have more energy and zest for sex?

Dave recalls his first on-the-pump sexual experience. "I was with a girl I had really liked for a long time. She was so cool about the pump and even wanted me to show her how to detach it. She kind of made it into foreplay. It was great sex because I wasn't worried about problems with my blood sugar or staying hard. I told her how I had to check my blood sugar after sex, and she totally reminded me to do it," he recalls.

I had a similar positive experience in opening up about the pump. I had gone out on one date with the man who is now my husband before going on the pump. All through dinner I kept thinking, "Sure, he likes me now . . . but wait until he finds out I'm about to become the bionic insulin pump woman." Well, when I told him about going on the pump later over coffee, he could not be more excited for me. He offered to help and support me any way he could. At that moment,

I knew he was worth keeping! My going on the insulin pump did not inhibit the growth of our relationship, physically or emotionally.

TEEN TIPS

Dating and the Pump

WHILE YOU and your teenager need to discuss and decide together what is an appropriate age for sexual activity, you can be sure that he or she is already concerned about being attractive and finding a boyfriend or girlfriend.

Encourage your son or daughter to find friends and activities that make him or her feel good and foster self-esteem. When it comes to dating, let your teenagers know that anyone they go out with should feel comfortable with their diabetes. Anyone who isn't cool with pump therapy, no matter how cute or popular, isn't worth it.

I'm in a committed relationship, and my lover isn't worried about my getting the pump, but I'm a little concerned about the "nuts and bolts" of the whole thing. What exactly do you do with the pump during sex?

In terms of the "nitty-gritty" how-does-it-work, there are a few options for sex with the pump. Generally, it's okay to detach from the pump for thirty to forty minutes if your blood sugar is in the normal range. I always do a quick check as we're getting in the mood. If your sugar is running just a bit on the high side, you can also take a bolus to bring you back to an even place before detaching.

There are also ways to enjoy sex still keeping the pump connected. I've also found ways to clip the pump onto whatever lingerie I may be wearing. The leg garter also comes in handy. Sometimes, depending on how strenuous or active the sex is, I just leave the pump on the bed beside me. There is enough tubing that the pump will be safe and can lay out of harm's way. I haven't had an encounter in which the pump interfered with position!

Could going on pump therapy actually improve my sex life?

This is not a sex book, of course, and I won't offer any advice about sex itself. But I do know that whatever your sexual orientation and your current status as single, dating, multiple partners, or monogamous, your sex life will not be diminished in any way by going on the pump. Many women I've talked to who were single before starting the pump have reported that after starting on it, they attract new relationships. Let's face it: Feeling good about yourself and feeling as healthy as possible is sexy! If your partner is put off by the pump, then he or she is not worthy of the privilege of being intimate with you.

For men living with diabetes, impotence can be a very serious problem. Maintaining blood sugars in the normal range is the single best thing to do in order to avoid impotence. Going on insulin pump therapy has helped countless men who, no matter how hard they tried, were not previously able to achieve optimal blood sugar control. In this way, pump therapy is an answer to improving one's sex life.

I often get low blood sugars right after sex. How can pump therapy help with this most annoying problem?

Another bonus for pumping in the bedroom: an easy way to avoid those sex-induced hypoglycemia moments. For many people, a heavy dosage of lovemaking can get the heart rate going faster than a session on the treadmill. And, with long-acting insulin in your system, there's no way to avoid a low blood sugar without eating some carbohydrate snack before sex.

The physical activity of intercourse would often lead me to have a low blood sugar, either after or sometimes during sex. I could never gauge if I needed to eat something before sex, because, well . . . when something is spontaneous in nature, you can't judge your carbohydrate needs the same way you would for a workout. For me, this experience was pretty unpleasant, and needless to say didn't do a whole lot for my pleasure. When I started on pump therapy, I realized that by disconnecting from my pump or lowering my basal rate before sexual activity, I can always avoid hypoglycemia. And I didn't need to "eat a snack" at an awkward moment. Sex has been much more carefree and pleasant with this new freedom. Go pumping!

One word of caution about sex and the pump: Always remember to **reconnect** your pump before falling asleep. If you're having a late-night romance session and you've detached from your pump, you must—absolutely—not fall asleep in a state of bliss without reattaching. Because pump therapy relies on short-acting insulin, you don't have a reserve of long-acting insulin to rely on. Falling asleep without your pump could lead to an extremely high blood sugar, and even ketoacidosis. If you are someone who tends to get wiped out after having sex, ask your partner to remind you to reconnect. Some folks also set an alarm clock as lovemaking begins for an hour later, just in case they should need a back-up wake-up call.

TEN WAYS

TO ENJOY A HEALTHY
SEX LIFE ON THE PUMP

1. Good blood sugar control leads to a healthier, more energetic approach to all aspects of life.

2. For men dealing with impotence, pump therapy can lead them to the blood sugar control they need in order to achieve normal erections.

3. Talk honestly with your partner—even if it's your spouse of many years—about any feelings of awkwardness that may arise in sexual situations.

4. Find partners who are supportive and loving of the *whole* you—pump and all.

5. Check your blood sugar before sex and decide if you want to disconnect, take a bolus, lower your basal rate, etc.

6. Experiment with different lingerie or undergarments that look flattering with the pump.

7. Practice disconnecting your pump so that in the "moment" it's as easy and natural as can be. Let your partner practice too.

8. Keep a sense of humor—even with the pump, each and every sexual encounter won't be a magical moment. Laugh it off and look forward to the next time!

9. Check your blood sugar after sex and make adjustments as needed.

10. *Do not* fall asleep after sex without reconnecting. Set an alarm as needed and/or train your partner to wake you up should you fall asleep.

EIGHT

Money Makes
the World Go Round . . .

AH, MONEY, SOMETHING that can be even scarier than sex! You may have heard about how expensive the insulin pump is (roughly $5,000 for the pump and up to $150 to 300 per month for pump supplies). When I realized I was walking around with something on my belt worth more money than my used Honda, I was shocked! Fortunately, my insurance company paid the entire cost of the pump and for my needed supplies.

People who feel a bit anxious about using such an expensive piece of medical equipment, take note: Your insulin pump can be covered by a renter's or homeowner's insurance policy. Insurance companies will issue a special floater, as they would for an expensive piece of jewelry.

It seems like all I do is fight with my insurance company over how many blood sugar test strips I can get a month. I don't know if I have the energy to take on another battle with pump supplies.

Again: Knowledge is power. The bureaucracy of managed health care can be mind-boggling; still, with a little effort, you should be able to break through the red tape and reach a real live person. Ask to speak with a manager or head of department; find out exactly what your insurance will cover. More and more, many American states are mandating coverage for diabetes supplies and this will cover the insulin pump and pump supplies. Fortunately, Medicare now covers the cost of the insulin pump for people with type 1 diabetes.

What is even better is that the major pump manufacturers—Animas, Disetronic, Medtronic MiniMed, and Sooil—all have trained professionals on their staff, whose entire job is to advocate for you to your insurance company. They know which companies are easy to deal with, which are more difficult, and how to convince them that the insulin pump is a medical necessity for you. Slowly, insurance companies are realizing that in the long run, they will save tremendous amounts of money if people with diabetes can achieve optimal blood sugar control and so avoid complications. As stated, insulin pump therapy has proven to be key in tight control.

Kathy Kochan remembers that when she ordered her insulin pump six years ago, it took a good six months for her to get insurance approval. "I was ready to go, but I had to sit around and wait for the insurance to get straightened out," she recalls. Fortunately, most pump companies are able to work with insurance companies so that there is only a two- to three-week delay from the time you make your decision to pump.

Interestingly enough, there appears to be a correlation between people living in countries with managed health care, in which money is not an issue around supplies, and good diabetes control. Disetronic is a Swiss-based company with large markets in Western Europe. Their studies show that people living in Scandanavia, the Netherlands, Germany, and France—for whom getting on pump therapy involves very little red tape—have an 85 percent better rate of optimal diabetes control than people living with diabetes in the United States. Medtronic MiniMed has a majority share of the insulin pump market in such countries as Italy and Israel, and finds the same to be true there. For being the "richest" country in the world, the United

States has much to learn about providing adequate health care for all. Sadly, in developing countries with very poor health care systems, pump therapy is virtually nonexistent in the present time.

By the way, if you are a citizen of the United Kingdom and are concerned about medical coverage for your pump, check out the Web site www.insulin-pumpers.org.uk. This site includes lots of good information about how to best work with the health care system there, to insure financing of your pump.

I've been approved by my insurance to get started on a pump. But I'm worried that my insurance will give me problems about the monthly supplies, which seem pretty hefty. And what if I change jobs. What then?

There is no doubt that for most American citizens, dealing with insurance issues can create many headaches. When it comes to pump therapy, there may be problems that arise.

Mort Waldbaum is now well adjusted to life with the pump but is still struggling with Medicare. "Medicare allows me thirty infusion sets for ninety days," Mort explains. "But I'm on a heart defibrilator that takes up room where my insertion sites would be. When I'm looking for a good site, I could go through 2 to 3 sets each time I try to insert one. And Medicare won't pay the difference." Especially for senior citizens living on a fixed income, this kind of challenge can be daunting.

Changing jobs can also cause insurance nightmares. Carys Price recalls the outcome of a job change. "It was a major headache. Getting my pump supplies with my new insurance became the biggest headache in the world. I would order supplies from one of these big companies, and wait and wait. Where are these people? When you call and leave them a message, they don't call back," she reports.

Eventually, Carys got her annoying insurance situation straightened out, but not without a good deal of energy and effort. I've gone through three insurance changes during my three and a half years on the pump, and fortunately, I can't complain. Again, since the pump companies have professionals on board who will do the legwork for you, I give it over to them and let them handle it. I've had success every time.

One more bit of good news: Insulin pumps are constantly improving with better technology, and most insurance companies will approve you for a brand-new insulin pump every four to five years. Again, check with your company to find out their policy on upgrading pumps.

My doctor wants me to go on an insulin pump, but my husband recently got laid off from his job and we're going to lose our health care coverage. I don't know when we'll get new insurance. How can I consider taking my doctor's advice?

For people without insurance or with plans with inadequate coverage, don't despair. Contact your local ADA and JDRF and find out about financial assistance for pump users. Also, both the Lions Club and the Rotary Club, in certain areas, offer scholarships to help pay for pumps. In Canada, a special charity called S.U.G.A.R. helps people pay for pumps; you can find them on-line at www.sugarcharity.org.

I've heard about people without health insurance who have done fund-raisers to help earn money to buy a pump. At some point or another, most of us have to ask for help with something in our lives. You may be surprised by how many people would be willing to donate a few dollars to the cost of your pump. I know how hard it is to ask for help. But above everything—even your pride—should be concern for your health.

You may also want to explore getting a DANA pump from Sooil, a Korea-based pump manufacturer. Sooil has recently opened their market to the United States and Western Europe, and is willing to offer a special payment plan through some distributors. Go to www.danapumps.com for more information.

But suppose my pump just breaks one day, or what if I have a freak accident? Is my insurance going to pay for another pump?

Should anything happen to your pump, you have no worries. All of the major pump companies offer a four-year warranty, which means that they will replace your pump at no cost to you. Remember, after four years you are eligible for a pump upgrade, so once you get your new pump, you will then have a new four-year warranty.

Talk with the manufacturer of the pump you are interested in purchasing and become clear on its policy. All of the companies will strive to replace your pump within twenty-four hours; some will even have a customer service representative drive a pump out to you so that your wait is only a few hours long. Interestingly enough, Disetronic's top-selling pump is still the H-Tron Plus, even though a newer model, the D-Tron, comes with more sophisticated features. The reason for the H-Tron's popularity is that when you order one, you receive *two* pumps automatically, so you would never have to switch back to injection therapy (even for a few hours) if you lost or broke your pump. Other companies, such as Animas, will lend you a second pump if you plan to travel overseas or have a child going away to camp. When you (or your child) return from wherever it is, you simply have to return the back-up pump to them. That's what I call service!

TOP TEN

Ways to Deal with Money and Insurance
Issues While Pumping

1. Educate thyself: These issues will be less scary if you know exactly where you stand with your health coverage.

2. Pick a pump company and let the insurance department handle negotiating for you.

3. Make sure your doctor is on board and is willing to write a letter of medical necessity for you. Also, keep good blood glucose logs to prove to the insurance company that you need a pump.

4. If you are on Medicaid or Medicare, you can pursue full coverage of your insulin pump.

5. If you want extra peace of mind, you can take out an insurance policy on your pump.

6. Be patient: Even once you've made your decision to choose pump therapy, dealing with your insurance company can delay your getting started for a few weeks.

7. If you are already pumping, find out when you are eligible for a replacement pump.

8. If you do not have insurance or adequate coverage, plan to fund-raise for your pump.

9. Again, keep a sense of humor: Laughing at the red tape of insurance companies is healthier than getting stressed out by them!

10. Donate money to your local ADA or JDRF chapter to establish a fund for insulin pumpers in need.

NINE

Inconvenience, or How Much More Do I Need to Schlepp?

Let's FACE IT—anyone with diabetes is a schlepper—someone who's always carrying extra things around with them. You know the routine; forget American Express, don't leave home without your insulin, syringes, blood sugar meter, strips, glucose, glycagon, prescriptions for insulin, or syringes. The thought of carrying even more "stuff" around can be daunting!

All right, lay it on me. What else do I need to keep with me if I go on this pump thing?

Going on the pump means being prepared to deal with its mechanical issues at any moment, and, yes, that means you'll have to keep a few more supplies with you. Pump batteries (they're very small), are absolutely necessary, as are infusion sets and insulin cartridges. The way I look at it, going on the pump is a great excuse to buy that new purse, backpack, attaché, etc. that you've been eyeing!

We all have stories about our stupidity when we were caught without the needed supplies. Fred (my husband) and I had a dinner date a few weeks after I went on the pump. We met at his apartment and walked a few blocks to a Greek restaurant. I wasn't in the mood to schlepp my purse and I knew we'd be gone for just an hour or two and then would return to his place. I put my money and keys in my pocket and we went out the door. We were seated at a table and ordered. Music was playing and I felt so happy to be getting adjusted to my pump and to be out to dinner with this wonderful man. Just as our dinner arrived, my pump started beeping: low battery! If I had had my purse with me, I could have changed the battery in a minute or two, right at the table. But no! We left the restaurant, walked home, I changed the battery, and we walked back to dinner. The waiter was very nice and kept our food hot; still, it was an unnecessary interruption that could have easily been prevented.

For parents of children on the pump, there is, of course, an extra imperative to make sure your child is well supplied at school and wherever he or she goes. For teenagers, this minor hassle can become a major problem. Some teens feel it's not "cool" to carry their supplies around, and "accidentally" forget them at home. It is critical that teenagers understand the importance of carrying their pump and other diabetes supplies with them always, before they are permitted to go on the pump. Usually finding the right backpack or bag to tuck supplies away in, unnoticed, can remedy the "stigma" of carrying extra stuff.

For people who spend equal time at home and at the office, play it safe and keep an extra infusion set and batteries in your desk drawer. Should you accidentally forget to schlepp your diabetes supplies on the day you need them most, your back-up set will be waiting for you.

Why would I need to carry syringes and vials of insulin if I'm using the pump? Can't I just keep an extra insulin cartridge on me?

Going on the insulin pump means saying good-bye to your old relationship with your syringes, or insulin pen. No more daily, multiple injections. But, think of these devices as an old friend that you may go visit every once in a while.

As mechanically advanced as insulin pumps are today, they can still have mechanical glitches from time to time . . . and you don't want to get stuck in a pump meltdown moment without a back-up source for insulin. Occasionally, strange things happen with pumps and they may (again, very rarely) shut down.

Even more commonly, you may be having trouble with an infusion site that is causing your insulin to not be properly absorbed. This can happen when an infusion site hits a blood vessel, for example. By the time you check your blood sugar, take a bolus of insulin, let some time go by, check again, and realize that your sugar is not coming down and there may be some kind of problem with your pump, your sugar could have risen quite high. Rather than stop and change your infusion site, it is recommended to take short-acting insulin through an injection, so it gets into your system immediately. As you begin to feel better, you can then change your infusion site. You will be happy to have your old friend, the syringe, handy for that moment!

WORD TO THE WISE

Carrying Insulin

YOU CONSIDER yourself to be prepared for any situation. You've got all you need to pump insulin with you, plus back-up insulin and syringes. But how long, exactly, have you been carrying around that vial of insulin? Weeks? Months? Years?

Remember that unrefrigerated insulin, especially if it's been in a hot purse or backpack, has an average shelf life of six months. While you're at it, check the expiration date on your glycagon kit. Whoops!

You may want to mark your calendar or PalmPilot with a six-month reminder to check on the freshness of your diabetes supplies. Couldn't hurt!

And if you should be caught in a situation in which you desperately need an insulin syringe, you can go into a pharmacy and ask for one. Show them a vial of insulin and your medical tag, and they should give you one syringe to get you by.

I hate wearing a medical tag, but my doctor said he won't prescribe a pump for me unless I promise to wear one. I've never had a problem where I've needed help. What's the big deal?

For any of us living with diabetes, as scary as this idea may be, we have no choice but to prepare for the fact that our blood sugar could rise or fall to dangerous levels, and that we would need immediate medical assistance. Wearing a medical alert bracelet or necklace must be viewed as just another thing we have to schlepp wherever we go. Medic Alert is the oldest and most reliable medical tag company in the United States. You can have printed on your tag "Insulin Dependent Diabetes, Wears Pump."

Sadly, many physicians and nursing staffs are not as familiar with insulin pump therapy as they should be. In the unfortunate case that you or someone you love with an insulin pump were in an automobile accident and were unconscious, the emergency room staff may have no idea of how to deal with a pump . . . or even what it is! While this sorry state of medical education is changing, we must advocate and protect ourselves. A Medic Alert necklace means that your physician (and loved ones) will be contacted immediately, and can give the attending physicians instructions about how to deal with your diabetes care. A tiny piece of jewelry can offer so much peace of mind.

Keep all of your pump supplies with you always—a little schlepping goes a long, long way.

TEN PUMP SUPPLIES
to Keep with You
Wherever You Go!

1. Extra infusion sets

2. Pump batteries

3. Insulin cartridges/reservoirs

4. Insulin syringes

5. Short-acting and long-acting insulin

6. Blood sugar meter and strips

7. Glucose tablets or something to eat for hypoglycemia

8. Emergency glucagon kit

9. Medic Alert necklace or bracelet

10. Prescriptions for insulin and syringes (just in case)

TEN

The Mechanics of the Pump, or, "But I Can't Even Program My VCR!"

ONCE I GOT over my emotional hurdles and felt pretty ready to start pumping, I still had one significant fear: figuring out the mechanics of the thing. Honestly, I really can't program my VCR. I voiced these concerns to Joyce Chub, my pump representative from Disetronic. "You'll do fine," she'd tell me. "Anyone can do it." All right, I thought, I'll try it. I'll try.

When Joyce came over to my apartment for my first pump lesson, I expressed my concern about the mechanics of the thing. "Gabrielle," she said, "children can work the pump. Senior citizens. People who are blind." Joyce showed me the simple procedures of putting in an insulin cartridge, changing batteries, changing the pump from "pumping" to "stopping." I tried to do what she showed me on my own. "Wow," Joyce said. "You're really not mechanical, are you?"

I'm a "low-tech" person and don't mind drawing insulin into a syringe. What exactly am I going to need to learn to go on the insulin pump?

I was very pleased to find out that I'm not the only person in the world who was intimidated about learning the mechanics of the pump. Sonia Seifert recalls her first thoughts about working with a pump, "I'm sixty-five years old and not computer comfortable. What if I press the wrong buttons and give myself too much insulin?" Sonia overcame her fears by working with her diabetes educator, Gary Scheiner (who wrote the foreword to this book), whom she could call even after she had started pumping if she had a mechanical question. Sonia, like many new pumpers, also took advantage of calling her company's toll-free number, at which a technician can always take you through a basic procedure like changing batteries, should you forget. I called my pump's 800 number repeatedly during my first few weeks of pumping, when I needed reassurance about working with the pump.

What I don't like about the insulin pump is that it is a machine—what if it "melts down" just like my computer does from time to time? What then?

In the early, experimental days of pump therapy, these fears would be quite well founded. Yerachmiel Altman remembers how with his first insulin pump there were no alarms to indicate mechanical errors. Sometimes his pump would deliver thirty to forty units of insulin . . . and he would need to eat to cover it all in order to avoid a severe hypoglycemic reaction.

Fortunately, technology has come a long, long way and today's pumps are really engineering marvels. They are equipped with alarms that will alert you of mechanical problems, and they have built-in protective devices such as letting you bolus only so much insulin at once. With all of that taken into consideration, it is still critical to remember that you, the pump user, must be "in control" of this little machine at all times. It is your responsibility to check your blood sugars regularly, to change your infusion sights every 2 to 3 days, to keep your insulin cartridges full. The mechanics of the pump should work very smoothly if you are doing the ongoing maintenance that the pump requires.

"It's really amazing how simple the mechanics of the thing are," marvels Gary Russell, president of Fifty50 food products for people with diabetes and himself a pump user for four years. "It's a double screw, a small computer, and some batteries!"

Quite amazing—when we stop and consider how great an impact this small machine can have on our health, and on our lives.

KIDS' CORNER

The Computer Generation

FOR MOST children growing up today, mastering the mechanics of the pump is a piece of cake. They know better than their parents—and definitely their grandparents—how to use GameBoys, computers, DVD players, etc. Computerized gadgets are just part of their lives.

For many kids, learning the mechanics of the pump can be one of the "coolest" parts about choosing pump therapy. Showing friends or relatives their expertise at changing batteries or infusion sites can boost the pumping kid's self-esteem.

Parents should remember that while kids have an easy time with the pump's mechanics, they may have a harder time dealing with the responsibility that the pump requires, such as staying regular with changing infusion sites. That's where Mom or Dad can be most helpful in giving gentle reminders, until the life lesson of taking responsibility is mastered too.

I'm willing to try to learn the "mechanics" of the pump . . . but where do I begin?

When you are choosing a specific pump manufacturer, I recommend that you make sure that a customer service representative is available to train you one-on-one, and that you will be able to call this person as needed with your questions. Having my pump rep available to do a training, in my home, helped me learn the basics in a fairly short amount of time.

Yes . . . with a little persistence and determination, nonmechanical me got the hang of working the pump within a few days. It took me some serious practice, which I recommend for every pump user before starting to actually pump insulin. Now I don't even think about the mechanics of the pump . . . it's easy-peasy stuff! But about my VCR . . .

Part of getting comfortable with the mechanics of the pump will also come from experience—you'll learn tricks as you go along. Sonia remembers that the most stressful part of working with the pump was changing infusion sites. On the days she needed to change them, she would do it in the morning as she was busy getting ready for work. "It was stressful because I didn't have a lot of time, and the more I rushed, it was harder to do," she says. After speaking with Gary Scheiner, her educator, about this problem, Sonia realized that she didn't have to change her infusion sites in the morning. "Just doing it in the evening, when I was more relaxed, made the whole thing so much easier," she explains. You will find your tricks, with experience, to make the simple mechanics of the pump work best for you.

TEN WAYS

TO MASTER THE MECHANICS
OF THE PUMP

1. Watch the videos your pump manufacturer produces that show the step-by-step instructions for working the buttons on the pump, changing batteries, etc. Pause on the steps that seem more complicated, rewind, and watch again.

2. Visit a pump support group and observe people using their insulin pumps.

3. Before you start to use your pump, practice, practice, practice!

4. Call the 800 number on your pump when in doubt.

5. Have a contact person you can call when you're really flustered—your pump rep, educator, or another insulin pumper.

6. Try to do any mechanical things that are in your control—changing cartridges, infusion sets, etc.—when you are relaxed and can take your time.

7. Have a family member or close friend learn the mechanics along with you so that they can be a support too.

8. Keep the card your pump company will give you, outlining what all of the alarm signals mean, with you at all times, so that you will know what to do should an alarm go off.

9. Feel confident—today's pumps are designed to protect you.

10. Be patient—learning new things takes a different amount of time for each individual.

ELEVEN

Exercise with the Pump

FOR MOST OF us, regular exercise is an important part of our diabetes control and our healthy lifestyle. Yet, for people with diabetes, it can be a struggle to optimally control blood sugar while exercising. Another clear advantage of pump therapy is that it allows you to more easily regulate your blood sugars while running, walking, swimming, etc. You just need to spend some time figuring out what adjustments work best for you during exercise. According to a recent study, "Pumping Insulin During Exercise," "The insulin regimen that makes an exercising diabetic individual's response closest to normal is continuous subcutaneous insulin infusion (CSII) therapy, also called insulin pump therapy." With experience and proper blood sugar testing, the pump user can adjust the fast-acting insulin in a pump, so that physiological response to exercise is more similar to a nondiabetic individual's. In other words, without the peaks and sometimes unpredictable effects of long-acting insulin, a pump user can lower basal rates, so that like in a nondiabetic individual, only a small amount of insulin is released during exercise.

When you first begin pumping, you will need to experiment a bit with how much to adjust your basal rates. The intensity and type of your workout will call for specific adjustments. You will need to stop and test your sugars while you are working out to determine whether you need to raise or lower your basal rates. But within a short time you will learn where you need to set your basal rate for a thirty-minute walk, and you'll be able to get through your workout with the confidence of knowing that your sugar is not going to suddenly drop too low.

How do I figure out how to set my basal rates correctly for working out?

Carys Price is a very active person who often participates in ten-mile runs. When she first started pumping, she patiently used trial and error to figure out how to set her basal rates. "I actually found that when doing a ten-mile run, I could take my pump off altogether. If I started just a bit high, like around 200, I would finish the run at 95," she explains. Monitoring your blood sugars post-exercise is also critical in determining how long you may need to keep basal rates lowered.

Kim Seeley is a personal trainer and fitness competitor who tests her blood sugar an hour before exercising, right before starting, sometime during, right after, and two hours after, so that she can make adjustments as needed. Kim works out intensely with weights, and has found that that type of anaerobic exercise can make her blood sugars skyrocket, and she needs to take an additional bolus. Kim has created her optimal workout routine by doing weight training first, followed by cardio activity, which brings her sugars down. Kim is an active member of the national Diabetes Exercise and Sports Association (which you can find out more about on-line at www.diabetes-exercise.org) and is continually fine-tuning the metabolic effects of working out. She knows that the insulin pump is the best way for her, as a diabetic, to achieve her personal fitness goals. Even for those of us who are noncompetitive athletes, the benefits of using a pump to control blood sugars during exercise is a huge payoff. Kathy Kochan has actually permanently set her morning basal rates in response to her morning workout. "I get up and exercise at the same time every day, seven days a week," Kathy explains. "So my basal rate is set at a very low amount, so that I can exercise without getting low."

If your exercise routine is not set, don't despair: Setting your basal rate at a temporary lower rate will work just fine. Another benefit of being able to do so means that you may not need a carbohydrate snack before exercising (unless your blood sugar is under 100 mg/dL when you start). Again, the type of exercise you will be doing, as well as the intensity of the workout, will determine how you set your basal rate and if you need a snack.

When I first was pumping, I had been in a routine of jogging three times a week for thirty minutes or so. I always checked my blood sugar before going, and if it was under 130, I ate some kind of snack. It always annoyed me that I had to eat extra calories before going to burn them off . . . but if I didn't, I would usually get low. While I jogged, I carried glucose tabs with me and often halfway through would need to eat one or two of them because I felt a little shaky. Still, I loved jogging and knew it was ultimately beneficial for my mental and physical health. I was terrified to start jogging after going on the pump. Ned Weiss, my endocrinologist, kept telling me to experiment—lower my basal rates, take my monitor with me, test along the way, and make any adjustments needed. Easy for him to say! I had visions of my sugar going so low, I would pass out along the road. I didn't want to ask a friend to jog with me because I felt bad that I'd slow them down when I had to stop and test. Stubborn me!

Finally, I couldn't stand not running, so I gave it a try. My blood sugar was 150 before I started. I decreased my basal rates by 30 percent before I began my jog. I didn't eat a snack. I stopped and tested halfway through. My blood sugar was 98. I decreased again, now giving myself just 40 percent of my usual basal rate. I got home and cooled down. My blood sugar was 81. I felt fantastic! I hadn't needed a snack and could adjust my insulin with the push of a button! Exercising was actually easier with the pump—wow!

Matthew Lore, my publisher at Marlowe & Company, is a relatively new pump user, and was also astounded by his ability to keep his blood sugars stabilized while exercising intensely. "Recently, I rode my bike for thirty minutes from my office to Lincoln Center for a performance of the New York City Opera. I was 122 when I started the ride, and lowered by basal rate to .2 and kept it there for the duration of the performance. I was 109 at intermission. Before jumping back on my bike for the forty-minute ride home later, I ate half a banana. When I got home, I checked my sugar and it was 100," he marveled.

WORD TO THE WISE

Keep Good Records!

WHILE MANY of us keep good records of our blood sugars and the food we eat, fewer of us regularly record our exercise. When adjusting to pump therapy, it is critical to keep good data about the time of day and duration of your exercise, and how you adjusted your basal rates before, during, and after your workout.

Amazingly, you may find that physical activity that you don't think of as "exercise" may require you to lower your basal rates. Some pump users report that they need to adjust their basals during housecleaning, especially if they're going up and down stairs doing laundry, or heavy vacuuming.

Look at your exercise data with your physician or educator to best determine how to adjust your basal rates. No physical activity is too strenuous or rigorous for you as long as you have proper planning to insure tight blood sugar control.

Different types of exercise may call for various adjustments with the pump. I have been a yoga enthusiast for several years and was very concerned about how my pump might interfere with performing the various postures that form Hatha yoga. I'm talking about inversions like shoulder stands and headstands! I spoke with my yoga teacher before returning to class with my pump. She basically encouraged me to try yoga with the pump, leave class and test when needed, do what I needed to do. Essentially, the pump doesn't interfere in any way with my yoga practice, and I've learned how much I need to decrease my basal rates for a strenuous yoga session. Interestingly, Matthew Lore reports that his biggest challenge so far is dealing with his

Bikram-style yoga classes, in which yoga poses are done in a 110-degree room at 60 percent humidity. The heat and exertion of the exercise mean that his blood sugar can drop 100 plus points over the course of the exercise. Like Carys during her runs, Matthew has found out that starting his workout just a bit high allows him to finish within a normal blood sugar range.

SUCCESS STORIES

Kim Seeley— fitness competitor

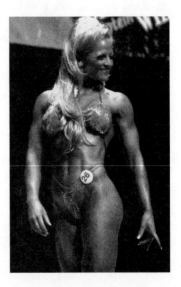

KIM REMEMBERS always enjoying athletics as a youth . . . and showed so much promise that at age twelve, the high school track and field coach took notice of her abilities and invited her to run drills against his high school athletes. He hoped that when track season came around, Kim would join them for full training. Before that time arrived, Kim became very ill, losing twenty pounds, and eventually collapsed one day walking home from the school bus. She was thirteen years old then, and diagnosed with type 1 diabetes.

Her hometown was small and lacked much medical support. Her family doctor told her that athletics would be difficult to deal with, and that she should focus on controlling her diabetes instead. Kim quit sports, and recalls all through high school watching the dancers dance, the runners run . . . all the while feeling bitter that she had been told not to join in.

Years later, as an adult, Kim joined a gym and began working out. At age twenty-seven, she hired a personal trainer and fell in love with muscle building. Two years later, after reading an article about fitness competition, Kim felt intrigued and decided to compete in her first show. She learned from that first experience, and became determined not to quit. Kim has held such impressive honors as winning first place in the 2002 Ms. Fitness Midwest competition, first place in the 2001 Ms. Fitness Rocky Mountain State, and being selected for a $5,000 scholarship (awarded to three athletes nationwide) for the 2001 Lifescan Athletic Achievement Award. Kim feels that being on the insulin pump puts her on an equal playing field with her competitors and that she could not get such a tight grip on diabetes control with injections. Kim still struggles with highs and lows, needing to cut back and increase insulin levels according to when she is in training/competition seasons.

Where does Kim's motivation come from? "There is nothing I can do about having diabetes; however, there is a lot I can do with my attitude about life with it. I can whine and cry about something out of my control . . . or I can just go for it. Either way, diabetes is still there. I have strength because I accept what I have to live with but have total focus on working on those things in life that can be changed. I'm strong because I know the difference," she explains.

Kim acknowledges that each human being—including her fitness competitors—face challenges, and that for her, diabetes is her unique challenge. The young girl who was told to give up athletics now knows that it is up to her to choose whether she quits or goes for her dreams. Diabetes, she says, is irrelevant.

I play football and basketball in my high school's varsity league. Is it safe for me to wear a pump during games?

Pumping insulin can even be effective for people playing high-physical-contact sports, like football and hockey. While some doctors okay using the pump under protective gear, others recommend that athletes take the pump off before a practice or game. With frequent blood sugar monitoring, the athlete can take an injection of insulin if his or her blood sugar starts to go high. Talk with your doctor or educator to see what he or she recommends; your pump company may also have tips from other users who play contact sports.

Pumping insulin sounds like such a great way to go for an exercise enthusiast like me. Are there any drawbacks to exercising with the pump?

People who are exercising with an insulin pump do need to be aware of a few potential challenges. First and foremost, check your insertion site while exercising to make sure that it hasn't been displaced in any way. If strenuous exercise causes the insertion site to come loose, insulin delivery will be stopped.

Some people who sweat excessively during exercise have reported that their sweating actually causes the insertion site to come loose. If you are a heavy sweater, you may want to use additional adhesive tape to keep your site in place. Also, antiperspirant can be applied to the skin where you will be placing your insertion site.

It is critical to remember that if your blood sugar is 250mg/dL or over, you must check for ketones before exercising. At that high level, exercise can actually cause your blood sugar to go higher, putting you in the danger zone. If ketones are present, you need to take a bolus of insulin and drink plenty of water. Wait until your blood sugar has stabilized before exercising. Keep in mind that even short-acting insulin remains in your system for three to four hours, so if you overbolus, you could be in danger of getting a low blood sugar.

As always, remember that extreme heat or cold can cause insulin to degrade and lose its effectiveness. If you have been exercising in extreme heat or cold, monitor your blood sugars closely. You may need to replace your damaged insulin cartridge with a fresh one.

These precautions aside, most pump users report that their newfound ease in exercising is one of the biggest payoffs of insulin pumping. Whether you hike, swim, cross-country ski, lift weights, or take part in competitive sports, your insulin pump will allow you to work out and achieve optimal blood sugar control.

TEN TIPS

1. Test, test, test! Before, during, and after. Taking the time to test your blood sugar is your best insurance for keeping your sugar in a normal range.

2. Be willing to experiment. You may not set your basal rates just right the first (or second or third) time you work out . . . but you'll get there.

3. Drink plenty of water while working out, to avoid dehydration.

4. Keep glucose tabs with you at all times, just in case.

5. Let your workout partners know about your pump and educate them about signs of hypoglycemia.

6. Remember that exercise can continue to lower your blood sugar for hours after your workout; you may need to keep your basal rate set at a lower rate post-workout. Especially if you exercise at night, a lower temporary basal rate can help prevent a low blood sugar reaction while you sleep.

7. If your blood sugar is under 70mg/dL before exercising, take some carbs to bring it up. If your sugar is over 250mg/dL, test for ketones and do not exercise if ketones are present.

8. If you are engaging in contact sports like football or hockey, you may want to remove your pump during the practice or game.

9. Check your insertion site, especially if you are sweating a great deal.

10. Experiment! Insulin pump therapy means that you can do any physical activity, with the proper adjustments, in a safe, healthy way.

TWELVE

Swimming, Water Sports, and Days at the Beach

IF YOU'RE A water-loving person like me, you may be concerned about how the insulin pump is going to interact with swimming. Many of today's pumps (such as Animas's R-1000, Disetronic's D-Tron, and Medtronic MiniMed's Paradigm pump) are waterproof and safe to use for all surface water activities, like swimming and diving.

However, because your pump is waterproof does not mean that you *have* to wear your pump for swimming; it just gives you that option. Most pump users I know find it most convenient to disconnect from their pumps for their daily shower or bath. And for an intense swim—just as with any other aerobic exercise—you may be able to disconnect your pump for best blood sugar results. Taking a small bolus if your blood sugar is a bit high before swimming can give you the insulin you need to sustain you while you swim. Also, be aware that certain infusion sets require a plug when going into the water, while others allow you to simply disconnect and take the plunge.

**But what about those lazy, hazy, crazy days of summer . . .
lounging by the pool and going in and out of the water
all day long?**

No problem—you can work with your pump in all situations, and spending long periods of time at the beach, a lake, or poolside is no obstacle. First of all, wearing the pump with a bathing suit is pretty simple for men—just clip it on your swim trunks, as you would do with a pair of shorts. For women, finding the right kind of suit is important. I went through some initial frustrations trying to clip my pump onto a one-piece suit. Not being a bikini model, I finally found a flattering two piece "tankini" that really does the trick for me. Easy to clip on, easy to disconnect.

Kim Seeley spends summer days at her family's lake. She brings a small cooler with her, so that when she detaches to go in the water, she can keep her pump in a safe place. She checks her blood sugar frequently during the day, and takes an injection if she needs some insulin to keep her sugars stable. Kim even water-skis with her water-proof pump attached.

Carys Price takes off her pump and puts it in a Ziploc bag with a cool pack when she spends time at the beach. She finds that she needs to check her blood sugar about every hour to make sure that her activity level (from swimming and walking) is keeping her blood sugar stable. She reconnects as needed, and takes a bolus if her sugars are running high.

WORD TO THE WISE

What About Sand in My Pump?

IF YOU plan to spend the day lounging at the beach and are worried about getting sand in your pump, don't fret. Small amounts of sand will not cause any kind of malfunction. However, if you are concerned that a lot of sand is getting in, or if you prefer to disconnect when at the beach, bring a cooler with you and keep your pump in it. Take a bolus before you detach, and check your blood sugar every forty-five to sixty minutes. You can reattach and bolus as needed, or simply bring along a syringe and vial of short-acting insulin. Many beachgoers find that the heat, combined with swimming, volleyball, walking, and other activities, requires less insulin than on a regular day.

If, on the other hand, you take your beach *lounging* seriously and consider proper beach activity to be reaching for the potato chip bag, make sure that if you detach, you are still getting enough insulin!

Remember to always keep your insulin in the shade, in a cool container. If your sugars are running high after your day by the pool, discard your insulin cartridge/reservoir and draw insulin from a fresh vial. It is always better to be safe than to risk taking sun-damaged insulin.

With a little extra planning, you will not have to give up the joy of swimming or any other water-related activity. Soon a day at the beach will feel like . . . well, a day at the beach!

One more tip for sea lovers: Even if you sport a waterproof pump, it's best to take it off before a jaunt in the ocean. Dave Cohen learned this lesson the hard way. "I was at the beach with some buddies and figured I'd leave my pump on while we rode waves," he says. "It was cool until I got smacked by this tremendous wave, and was swept into the undertow. I got up to the surface and saw my pump there floating beside me!" Dave was most fortunate to find his pump so easily, but his infusion set was ripped right off his skin. Fortunately, he had back-up supplies in a bag on the beach.

It's also important to remember that exposure to heat can affect your blood sugar—many people experience increased hypoglycemia when they're spending a day at the beach. With your pump, you can decrease your basal rates as needed to avoid getting low. Also, remember good common sense and keep reapplying sunscreen: A bad sunburn can affect your blood sugars too.

KID'S CORNER

Safe Splashing

WHEN KIDS go to the swimming pool, it can be hard to predict their activity level. Most times, they're not at the pool to do a session of laps, as adults may be. Kids jump in and out of the water, play games of Marco Polo, go down the sliding board countless times, engage in underwater races, etc.

Set the parameters of a swimming day with your son or daughter before you get to the pool. Make clear that they need to get out and test their blood sugar at the times you decide are appropriate. If they are not keeping their pump attached, they must be willing to reattach and bolus, or take a shot of insulin, as needed. Many parents have found that being disconnected from the pump for more than two hours can lead to a day of "chasing" blood sugars from high to low and back again.

Many swimming pool snack bars offer treats like ice cream and french fries; remind your kid to test and bolus as needed before eating. With a little forethought, a swim day can be enjoyable for everyone.

1. Check with your doctor—in most cases, it's just fine to disconnect for a shower or bath.

2. If you want to be able to swim with a pump on, check the various pump companies' models of waterproof pumps.

3. Find a bathing suit that will allow you to connect and disconnect easily.

4. Remember to take a cooler or cool pack along with you if you are planning to spend the day outdoors.

5. When you go into the ocean, always disconnect.

6. If you are going on vacation, make sure you have extra vials of insulin and syringes along with you in case of exposure to the sun.

7. Practice experimenting with lowering your basal rates to correspond with your swimming activity level.

8. Apply and reapply sunscreen—besides the pain of a sunburn, it can cause your blood sugar to rise.

9. Be aware that being in intense heat—and sweating profusely—can lower blood sugar levels in some people.

10. Relax and enjoy your day!

PART THREE

Preparing to Pump—
What You Need to Do
Before Your "Big Day"

ONCE YOU HAVE made the decision to go on the pump, you still
have some work to do before your actual day of connection. I have heard
many pump users who are parents compare this stage to setting up a
nursery for an expected newborn. You want to have everything in order
and ready to go, before those joyous—and initially overwhelming—days
of actually starting your pump therapy!

In the remaining time before you start with pump therapy, get a head
start on monitoring your blood sugars as closely as possible. Add a nighttime check, another midday check; check an hour after you eat. This
close monitoring will be essential in the first few days of your pump
therapy. If you start more frequent monitoring now, it will not only help
you control your blood sugars, it will also prepare you for a new, tighter

regime. The first few days of being on the pump can be overwhelming, to say the least. The total impact of the adjustment will be easier if you start your tight monitoring ahead of time.

If you are feeling nervous about starting the pump, you can practice being attached to it ahead of time. Your insulin pump rep can get your started using your pump with saline in the cartridges instead of insulin. You can do everything you would need to do while pumping, without a chance of doing any damage to your body. This "play pumping" can really help people who learn best by hands-on experience.

While most people don't feel that this step is necessary, it is recommended that you work with the pump off your body as much as you can. Insert batteries and practice going from stop to run and back again. Learn what all of the different functions are for, what different error alarms indicate. The more you practice with your pump before you get started, the easier your official beginning will be.

This section of the book outlines the other necessary steps to prepare you for successful control with your pump. Congratulations on your decision to choose pump therapy!

THIRTEEN

Which Pump to Choose?

ONCE YOU MAKE your decision to select pump therapy, you have another important choice to make: which insulin pump to choose. Pump users vary widely about their feelings toward the four major pump manufacturers—Animas, Disetronic, Medtronic MiniMed, and Sooil. If you log on to the insulin pumper's list serve (IP@insulin-pumpers.org), you can "listen in" on discussions that range from singing praises to lodging complaints about the pump companies. Some pumpers are very loyal to their specific brand and style of pump—others are always curious about what the other companies have to offer.

My doctor recommends a specific pump, but I've been doing a lot of research and don't understand why that pump is better than the others. Should I trust him?

In some cases, your doctor or diabetes educator may have one particular company that she favors, and will urge you to try that pump.

Generally, that's a good way to go—it means that she is most familiar with that pump's special features and can share that knowledge with you. However, if your doctor is guiding you toward a certain pump and you feel strongly that you want a different model, do not hesitate to speak up. The nuances among the insulin pumps out there are subtle enough that your doctor can master your pump's specific features right along with you.

It is easy to be influenced by a doctor or another pump user that you know, and decide to choose the pump brand and model that they suggest. Remember that their decision may be arbitrary and/or based on personal prejudice. For example, one endocrinologist I know favors Disetronic pumps because Disetronic is a Swiss company, and he considers the Swiss to make superior products. I recommend that you explore what each pump manufacturer has to offer, and make your decision based on knowledge.

How do I learn about what each pump has to offer?

If you are not certain about which pump to choose, spend some time on each Web site and/or order promotional material from each company. What is even more important is that you speak with a customer service representative from each company, so that you find a person that you feel comfortable working with. The chart I provide at the end of this chapter comparing the different pump features of many models out on the market today can help to guide your decision. But, ultimately choosing the best pump for you is an intuitive process. One of the insulin pumps will most likely "feel right" to you . . . and that should be your pump.

TEN WAYS

TO CHOOSE THE
RIGHT PUMP FOR YOU

1. Speak to your doctor or educator about her recommendations.

2. Review each company's Web site and promotional materials.

3. Speak with a customer service representative about the company and what support services it offers.

4. Place a call to the company's help line and see just how helpful they are! (No, you're not being a prankster—just conducting research!)

5. Talk with other pumpers (you can find them on the insulin pumper's list serve) about their experiences with each company.

6. Make a list of the features that are most important to you. Size? Waterproof? Years the company's been in business?

7. Review the Comparative Insulin Pump Chart on page 94 and see which pump meets most of your criteria.

8. Make sure you find out critical information about the company, such as their replacement policy, how long repairs take, length of time it takes for supplies to come, etc.

9. Take in all of this information, digest it, and let your answer come to you.

10. Remember, most insurance companies will allow you to get a new pump every four years, so you are not committing to this particular pump forever.

COMPARABLE INSULIN PUMP CHART

This chart compares the following current pump models on the market: Animas R-1000, Sooil (DANA) Diabecare II, Disetronic D-Tron, Disetronic H-Tron Plus, Medtronic MiniMed 508, and Medtronic MiniMed Paradigm. Thanks to Gary Scheiner, M.S., C.D.E., with whom this chart was created.

FEATURES OF ANIMAS R-1000
- Waterproof (up to 8 feet for 24 hours)
- DC motor (minimizes blockage in tubing)
- On-screen menus; no complicated button presses
- Basal delivery every 3 minutes regardless of basal rate (precise at low basal rates)
- .05-unit basal increments
- Starting basal rate 0.05
- Temporary basal rates set as percentage changes
- Slim design
- Rotating clip
- Recessed dedicated audio bolus button
- Low Cartridge warning alarm.
- Alarms explained onscreen
- Patented Rapid Occlusion detection with sensitivity option
- Silent rapid insulin delivery
- Lead screw sealed inside pump
- Multiple fashion covers with entire line of reusable stickers
- Rapid/quiet insulin delivery
- Uses over-the-counter batteries that last two to three months
- Non-Volatile RAM—Pump maintains its memory (for years) even if the batteries are removed
- 24-hour pump support with health care professionals

- Patient alerted for reordering of supplies
- Memory daily total past 255 daily and basal deliveries with date

    Past 255 alarms including full date and time

    Past 255 bolus amounts, including code for bolus type with date and time
- Tamper-resistant lock for children
- Thousands of safety checks hourly
- Insulin limit and auto-off safety options
- Holds 300 units insulin
- Weighs approx. 4 ounces
- 12-24-hour clock options
- Lighted screen
- Compatible with all infusion sets
- Replacement pump shipped overnight
- Company working to "close the loop"
- Accessories available
- 4-year warranty

Features of Sooil (DANA) Diabecare II

- Water resistant
- Swiss micro DC motor
- Temporary basal rates set as percentage changes
- Insulin limit and auto-off safety options
- Basal delivery every four minutes
- Low cartridge warnings
- Smallest full-feature pump on the market
- PIN access coding
- Cartridge can be visually inspected
- Lightest pump weight: 1.8 oz.
- Approx. 20 percent less expensive than other pumps
- Guided management offers 16 pre-programming options
- User-friendly ICON menu

- Extended bolus options
- Optional ability to pre-set meal-specific boluses
- Multiple basal rates and patterns
- Compatible with all infusion sets
- 24-hour phone support
- Battery life averages 3 months each
- Thousands of safety checks hourly
- Holds 300 units insulin
- Memory features include last 50 boluses, primes and daily totals, last 12 alarms—all time- and date-stamped
- Replacement pump shipped overnight
- Calculates daily totals
- Screen Sleep Mode—energy saver
- Audible tone (beep)
- Largest display screen of any pump available
- Comes with two leather cases, hard case, bra pouch, bathing bag, and other accessories
- Language options: English, Spanish, Chinese, Korean, Hebrew, Turkish
- Available in four colors
- 20 years in business; developed by Korean endocrinologist

FEATURES OF DISETRONIC D-TRON

- Watertight (up to 8 foot for 24 hours)
- Pre-filled cartridges
- DC motor (minimizes blockage in tubing)
- Basal delivery every 3 minutes (precise at low basal rates)
- Cartridge can be visually inspected
- Thousands of safety checks hourly
- Insulin limit and auto-off safety options
- Low cartridge warnings
- Holds 300 units insulin

- Weighs approx. 4 ounces
- 12- and 24-hour clock options
- Lighted screen
- Comes with spring-loaded clip case
- 7-point memory features
- Extended bolus options
- Multiple basal rates and patterns
- Compatible with all infusion sets
- 24-hour phone support
- Replacement pump shipped overnight
- Calculates daily totals
- Company working to "close the loop"
- Accessories available
- Patient alerted for reordering of supplies
- 4-year warranty
- Adjustable tone volume
- No plunge shift (insulin level stable with disconnection)
- 15 years in business
- Cartridge sealed securely inside pump
- Clock/messages always shown
- Vibrate option
- Temporary basal rates set as percentage changes
- Error messages explained on back of pump
- Rapid/quiet insulin delivery
- Rotating clip
- Silent mode option
- Easy switch to extended bolus
- Bolus up to 25 units

FEATURES OF DISETRONIC H-TRON PLUS

- Water resistant
- DC motor (minimizes blockage in tubing)
- Basal delivery every 3 minutes (precise at low basal rates)

- Cartridge can be visually inspected
- Thousands of safety checks hourly
- Insulin limit and auto-off safety options
- Low cartridge warnings
- Holds 300 units insulin
- Weighs approx. 4 ounces
- Memory features
- Extended bolus options
- Compatible with all infusion sets
- 24-hour phone support
- Patient alerted for reordering of supplies
- Replacement pump shipped overnight
- Comes with two pumps
- Calculates daily totals
- Company working to "close the loop"
- Accessories available
- 4-year warranty
- 15 years in business
- Cartridge sealed securely inside pump
- Temporary basal rates set as percentage changes
- Error messages explained on back of pump
- Rapid/quiet insulin delivery
- Bolus up to 25 units

FEATURES OF MEDTRONIC MINIMED 508

- Watertight (up to 8 feet for 24 hours)
- 20 years in pump business
- Child block option
- Thousands of safety checks hourly
- Insulin limit and auto-off safety options
- Low cartridge warnings
- Weighs approx. 3 ounces
- Holds 300 units of insulin
- 12- and 24-hour clock options

- Lighted screen
- Comes with spring-loaded clip
- Memory features
- Extended bolus options
- Multiple basal rates and patterns
- Compatible with all infusion sets
- 24-hour phone support
- Replacement pump shipped overnight
- Calculates daily totals
- Company working to "close the loop"
- Accessories available
- 4-year warranty
- Adjustable tone volume
- Beeperlike appearance
- Remote control
- Clock/messages always shown
- Alarm vibrate option
- Downloadable with meter (90 days of data)
- Compatible with U100, U50, and U40 insulin
- Diagnostic self-test function
- Automatic safety checks
- Normal, square wave, and dual wave bolus option
- Cartridge can be visually inspected
- Multilanguage capability
- Choice of four colors
- Priming function for accurate daily delivery tools
- Strong, easily removable clip
- Extensive data memory
- Bolus up to 25 units
- Large, easy-to-read screen

FEATURES OF MEDTRONIC MINIMED PARADIGM
- Watertight up to 8 feet for 24 hours
- 20 years in pump business

- Child block option
- Thousands of safety checks hourly
- Insulin limit and auto-off safety options
- Low cartridge warnings
- Weighs approx. 3 ounces
- 12- and 24-hour clock options
- Lighted screen
- Comes with spring-loaded clip
- Memory features
- Extended bolus options
- Multiple basal rates and patterns
- Compatible with all infusion sets
- 24-hour phone support
- Replacement pump shipped overnight
- Calculates daily totals
- Company working to "close the loop"
- Accessories available
- 4-year warranty
- Adjustable tone volume
- Beeper-like appearance
- Smallest full-featured pump
- E-Z Path Menu
- Silent motor, no clicking
- Remote control
- Clock/messages always shown
- Alarm vibrate option
- Uses single, over-the-counter batteries (AAA)
- Downloadable with meter (90 days of data)
- Compatible with U100 and U50 insulin
- Diagnostic self-test function
- Automatic safety checks
- Normal, square wave, and dual wave bolus option
- Cartridge can be visually inspected
- Multilanguage capability

- Choice of three colors
- Electronic priming
- Rotating clip-on-clip case
- Most extensive data memory
- Bolus up to 25 units
- Large, easy-to-read screen

FOURTEEN

Carbohydrate Counting, or What Evil Lies Within That Slice of Pizza?

WHEN I WAS first diagnosed with type 1 diabetes in 1982, people with diabetes were taught to use the exchange system to control their food intake. Within a few years of my diagnosis, I had internalized the exchanges and could eye food portions pretty easily. Of course, this led me to moments of "rationalized" cheating—sure that gigantic serving of pasta at a restaurant is the same size serving I eat at home!

For many of us, the exchange system was the best thing out there for balancing food, insulin, and activity. Many people with diabetes have "memorized" food exchanges and can manage the system fairly well.

I've had diabetes for thirty years. Please don't tell me that I need to learn a new way to deal with food and insulin!

The bad news is: Yes, if you are not carbohydrate counting already, you'll definitely need to learn how to do so. But the good news is most people find carb counting much easier to work with than the exchange system and are able to use carb counting and the pump to eat when and what they choose. Not a bad tradeoff!

Before considering the pump, I had not heard about carbohydrate counting as a way of monitoring food intake. But my endocrinologist explained that counting carbohydrates is how you determine the correct bolus to take to cover the food you're eating. The pump works on short-acting insulin—I use Humalog—so you can take only as much insulin as you need for what you're eating. No more eating to cover your insulin! In fact, you do not have to eat at all if you don't want to. Your ongoing basal rate will keep your blood sugars constantly in the healthy range; you bolus only when you eat carbohydrates. (See the Insulin/Carbohydrate Ratio Sheet on page 181 for more information).

For instance, if I am going to have a meal of broiled fish and salad, I may not need to take any bolus at all. By counting the carbohydrates in the food you're eating, you'll be able to determine exactly how much insulin to take. Liessa Demba eats very little carbohydrate in her diet, which consists largely of vegetables, fish and other lean meat, and fruit. She might eat a quarter cup of rice per meal or maybe some popcorn for a snack. "Because I eat so little carbohydrate, I can maintain excellent blood sugar control with mostly just my basal insulin. But if I do take a bolus and it's off, my blood sugars can go out of whack for hours," Liessa explains.

Don't despair: It takes some time and practice to get a sense of just how much insulin to bolus to cover the carbohydrates in the food you eat. When you are off, you will need to take a later "correction" bolus of insulin to bring your blood sugar back in balance.

WORD TO THE WISE

Two Numbers You Need to Know

WHEN YOU are first adjusting to pump therapy, your doctor or educator will help you to determine two critical numbers that will aid you in keeping tight blood sugar control as you learn to take bolus insulin:

1) How much one unit of insulin brings down your blood sugar when you're not eating, and 2) How much 1 gram of carbohydrate will raise your blood sugar.

While there are average numbers that work for many people, your numbers may be unique to you, based on such factors as your weight, insulin sensitivity, etc.

This example illustrates the importance of these numbers:

It's about half an hour before lunch, and you test your blood sugar to find it's 182 mg/dL. You want to start lunch in the healthy range, so you bolus .5 (½) unit of insulin *(your number*)*. At 12:15, your blood sugar is 120 mg/dL. You look at your lunch—soup, a salad with light dressing, a roll, and an orange. You calculate that you will be eating approximately 50 grams of carbohydrate. You know that you need 1 unit of insulin *(your number*)* for every 10 grams of carbohydrate. So, you bolus 5 units of insulin, and enjoy your lunch!

*Numbers are used for illustration purposes only; your doctor/educator will help you to find your most accurate numbers.

So how do I find out how much carbohydrate is in the food I eat?

Determining the exact carbohydrate count in your food and taking the correct bolus based on that determination takes some practice. Liessa's experiences with estimating boluses are not uncommon for new (and sometimes experienced) pumpers.

To begin with, when you first start pumping, you'll want to pick up a copy of a nutrition guide like *Bowes & Church's Food Values of Portions Commonly Used*. *Food Values* lists the carbohydrates in nearly every food under the sun—from fruits and veggies to brand-name products. I kept a pocket edition in my purse for quick estimations, anytime, anywhere, when I first started pumping insulin.

Cara Jennings found it easiest, when she made her transition to carbohydrate counting, to eat packaged foods that list the carb values right on the package. "I'd make a Lean Cuisine or Healthy Choice meal for dinner every night, and there it was right on the back of the package—how much carbohydrate was in my dinner.

That was a lot easier for me than making up a plate of rice and beans and figuring out the carbs. Of course, when I ate a piece of fruit, it seemed like no matter what, I was always off," she explains.

Again—carbohydrate counting requires patience, as well as trial and error. For example, a medium apple has 19 grams of carbohydrates. Well, say you've just brought a bushel of apples home—and they're all a bit different in size. Which one is the "medium"? "I had to be very patient with eating fruits and vegetables," Cara recalls. "On the exchange system, I counted an apple or an orange as one fruit! Now, if it was a really big piece of fruit, I needed to increase my bolus rate. It was a sort of 'mental' block I had to get through. And fruit cup—forget about it! I always took too much or too little insulin. I finally started catching on—you have to look at the fruit in the fruit cup to figure out how much to bolus. If grapes are in anything, forget about it—I always need more insulin than I think."

Cara's experiences point out a great advantage of pump therapy—by carefully taking bolus insulin, you can monitor how certain foods affect your blood sugars more than others. You will have the ability to precisely fine-tune your diet and insulin intake based on that knowledge. "I'm Italian, but I never cook red sauce," Kathy Kochan tells me. "It makes my blood sugars shoot right up. It's not worth it to me." In fact, Kathy eats more or less the same diet each day so that she doesn't have to worry about finding the exact bolus rate for a range of different foods. Many pump users do some variation on that style of eating—by repeating meals several times (and keeping good records), you can figure out exactly how much bolus you need to take. If you then repeat a few basic meals during the week, you can be sure to take the correct bolus for the carbs you are eating.

For parents of children starting pump therapy, be sure to include your kids in the carb counting process. Children can gain a sense of control over this new situation by being able to help mom and dad determine how much insulin they need. Parents can begin by sticking to their "usual" diet and then gradually adding new foods. Keeping a master list of carbohydrates in your family's most frequently eaten foods can shorten the learning curve for everyone.

I've heard a little about the glycemic index. What exactly is it, and will it help me to determine my bolus insulin?

The glycemic index (GI) is a ranking of foods based on their immediate effect on blood sugar levels. It can be a wonderful tool in helping you to calculate your bolus insulin needs. The GI is a reliable classification of foods that shows which carbohydrate foods break down quickly in the bloodstream (causing a sharp rise in blood sugar) and which foods break down slowly, causing a gradual rise in blood sugar. Foods that break down quickly have a high GI rating, while foods that break down slowly have a low GI rating.

In other words, different carbohydrates affect our blood sugars quite differently. What is especially helpful about the GI is that it dispels some of the formerly widely held beliefs about carbohydrates. For example, potatoes have a higher GI rating than does pasta. Tropical fruits like pineapple and bananas have a higher GI rating than "cool" fruits like apples and pears. This doesn't mean that you should give up potatoes and bananas; it simply means that the GI can also help you to determine how carbs will affect your blood sugar. Choosing carbohydrates that have a low GI rating can mean taking less insulin.

"All carbs are not created equal," laughs Gary Russell, "no matter what they say." Gary learned this reality (proven by the glycemic index) once he started pumping and saw how different varieties of bread affected his blood sugar, and consequently his insulin needs, in dramatically different ways.

When I started pumping, I wasn't very familiar with the GI, but I learned through trial and error that certain carbs made my blood sugars spike. I was startled by my intolerance of bagels—a favorite food. I had never realized how bagels made my blood sugars shoot up for hours after I ate one; I had always thought that midmorning highs meant I didn't have enough NPH insulin in my system. Instead, by bolusing for my bagels, I realized that it took an enormous amount of insulin for me to eat a bagel and keep my blood sugar in a normal range. I made a switch to breakfasts of multigrain cereal and yogurt, and save bagels for an occasional treat. The GI shows how the way that foods are processed, besides their basic content, can affect blood sugar rise. Bagels are highly processed foods, being made from refined flour and then both boiled and baked.

For more information on the glycemic index and how it relates to people with diabetes, check out *The Glucose Revolution Pocket Guide to Diabetes*. There is also a very helpful Web site, created by researchers at the University of Sydney, with a comprehensive guide to the glycemic index, www.glycemic index.com. There is new research coming out all of the time on GI, including a new table of values called the "glycemic load," which measures the glycemic index of a food multiplied by its carbohydrate content. Again, this information can help you to choose the healthiest foods for optimal blood sugar control.

KIDS' CORNER

The Birthday Party

DOESN'T IT seem like there are more children's birthday parties today than when we were growing up? It's normal for some kids to have a birthday party every weekend, sometimes twice in a weekend!

To keep your pumping kid's blood sugars under control, check in with host parents ahead of time and get a sense of what food will be served. Typical party fair is high-fat, high-carb stuff like pizza, chips, cake, and ice cream, that can make blood sugars rise for hours on end. Of course, some parties also involve lots of physical activity like games, swimming, roller skating, etc. that can help to lower blood sugar.

It will take some trial and error to determine the best strategy for birthday party days. Be patient; the first time (or two or three times) with parties and the pump may not work out perfectly. But with a little planning and good record keeping, the pump can allow your child to have her cake and eat it, too!

I'm always on the road and my job requires that I eat out in restaurants quite a bit. How am I going to figure out the carbs in everything I'm going to eat?

First off, remember that food is never a "precise" science, and many pump users tend to "estimate" carbohydrate values rather than keep a book or a scale with them at all times. The important thing is to test your blood sugar an hour after you eat, and take additional boluses as needed. If you've taken too much insulin, the pump allows you to temporarily lower your basal rate to compensate. Again—no more need to eat those extra calories to "cover" your insulin. Eating in restaurants can be challenging. There are often carbs hiding out where you may least expect it. Say you order grilled chicken breast for dinner, feeling confident that you're eating a low-carb meal. There may in fact be a good deal of sugar in the sauce that your chicken was marinated in, which in turn could raise your blood sugar. Again, test an hour after dinner and correct your bolus as needed. If you frequent certain restaurants repeatedly, make notes about how much you need to bolus for certain dishes. That way, you can order them again and know that you are taking the correct bolus.

"I always take a little more bolus when I eat out, but it always works out," says Kathy Kochan. "Restaurants just put more sugar in food than we realize. I'd rather take a bit more insulin than have my blood sugars go high."

Asian food in particular seems to have a mysterious effect on blood sugar. My first few times pumping and eating Chinese food were total disasters. Finally, I stopped eating rice and ate just meat and vegetables when I ate Chinese, and then I was fine. Like Kathy, I always bolus on the high side when I'm eating certain foods in a restaurant, like sushi. (Although I am sure to test my blood sugar before driving home, to make sure that I haven't way overbolused and am not in danger of getting low blood sugar.) I never knew why my sugars would go so high after eating sushi or white rice with Chinese food, until I learned from the glycemic index that white rice has a much higher GI rating than brown rice, which is what I normally cook at home.

So all I need to worry about is the carbohydrate value in food? Do I have to think about anything else?

Pumping insulin really allows you to be a scientist, determining how all food groups affect your insulin needs. Many pump users are shocked to learn about the lasting effects of high-fat food on their blood sugar. Dave Cohen, who eats his meals in his college dorm, was pretty shocked to discover what french fries and pizza were doing to his blood sugar.

"I would take what insulin bolus I thought was right and I'd be okay after dinner," he says. "Then I'd be studying a few hours later and start to feel like crap. I'd test my blood sugar and be like 300!" Dave discovered what many of us do—high-fat food has a definite impact on blood sugars. But not wanting to give up his favorite college staples, Dave and his doctor determined that he could raise his basal rate for three to four hours when eating pizza or the like, and that helped him to stay stable. He also checks his blood sugar two hours after eating (when his sugars would really start to rise) and takes an additional bolus as needed.

WORD TO THE WISE

Foods to Watch Out For!

WE ALL love to indulge from time to time. Just be aware that foods both high in fat and carbohydrate can make blood sugar levels rise for an extended time. Even if you check your sugar an hour after you eat, you may not catch the "major spike" yet. Test frequently and learn to adjust basal rates to compensate for high-fat, high-carb foods.

In a survey of pump users interviewed for this book, here is their list of top foods/meals to pay close attention to:

Pizza

Pancakes with butter and syrup

Breakfast buffets (especially those offering a big selection of muffins, pancakes, waffles, etc.)

Thanksgiving dinner

Movie theater popcorn (with butter, of course)

Ribs

Burger and fries

Carbohydrate counting helped me to realize that I was eating way too much high-fat, high-glycemic food and has helped me to create a much more nutritionally sound meal plan. While pump therapy could hypothetically allow a person to eat a total junk-food diet and maintain good blood sugar control, one of its great benefits is that it allows its user to create a diet based on healthy foods. We all have those foods that we just can't tolerate, and we also have foods that seem to help us magically keep our sugars stable. Living with diabetes means paying extra attention to our bodies, and giving them all of the vitamins and nutrients needed to create a healthy body, inside and out.

For people with diabetes, on the pump or not, carbohydrate counting (along with knowledge of the glycemic index) is a great way to learn how food and insulin interact. Your doctor, educator, or a nutritionist can help you learn the basics of carbohydrate counting. It is a very simple and straightforward way of monitoring your food intake.

What about counting carbs in alcohol? How do I figure out how much insulin to bolus for a drink?

If you want to include a moderate amount of alcohol in your meal plan, it is necessary to talk with your doctor or nutritionist about how to do so in a healthy way. Because having alcohol in your body can lower your blood sugar, it is critical that you learn how to bolus safely. Generally, it is recommended that you drink with a meal to avoid low blood sugar. Just as after any meal, if you're drinking, you need to be alert enough to test your blood sugar and make any necessary adjustments.

TEN TIPS
FOR CARB COUNTING

1. Buy a food values book (like *Bowes & Church's Food Values of Portions Commonly Used*) and keep it with you while you're learning to count carbs.

2. Keep good records so that you can recall how different foods affect your blood sugar.

3. Repeat meals, especially at first, so you can best determine correct basal rates.

4. Test an hour after eating and take a "correction" bolus of insulin as needed.

5. Start to eyeball food so that you know the difference between a small banana and a medium one, and how to adjust your bolus accordingly.

6. Pay attention to those "trouble" foods that make your sugars go up no matter what corrections you make.

7. When eating out, look for "hidden" sources of carbs, like sauces or gravy. Don't hesitate to ask your server for the exact ingredients listed in a dish.

8. Pay attention to food preparation—raw fruits and vegetables may have a different impact on your sugars than cooked ones, for example.

9. Remember Gary Russell's rule, "All carbs are not created equal." Stick to those carbs that you can best tolerate and are good for you—like multigrain breads, grains, and pastas.

10. Look out for high-fat foods or foods that are high in fat and carbohydrate, like good old pizza!

FIFTEEN

Your First Days on the Pump

NO MATTER WHAT you do to prepare yourself, the first few days of pumping will be challenging. You have so many new things to do: figure out the correct basal rates you need, adjust boluses correctly, insert your infusion sets, and more. Of course, you will have your doctor or educator there to guide you through the steps. But consider—how are you going to manage to deal with all these new things and still continue working, maintaining family responsibilities, going to school, etc.?

My doctor suggested that I go into the hospital for a few days while I get adjusted to my pump. I absolutely hate hospitals. Do I really need to be there?

The answer is—maybe. Health care professionals vary widely about the best way to get patients started on pump therapy. Their primary concern is, of course, for your health during this transition. Many physicians feel that the extreme change of going off long-acting insulin while trying to set a correct dosage of basal insulin requires a short hospital stay.

Doreen remembers how her two teenagers, Joe and Jessica, were transitioned onto pump therapy. "There we were, the two of them, Joe and Jessica, in the same hospital room. I'm a single parent, and this was the only way to make sure they got set up in a safe way. It was a little bit daunting for all of us, but the kids both took initiative," she recalls.

When I decided to get my pump, my doctor Ned Weiss suggested I be admitted to the hospital for a few days. At first I resisted. I hate hospitals and had managed to avoid them since my diagnosis when I was ten. I was really proud that in all those years since my diagnosis, I had never had to be hospitalized because of my diabetes. But Ned explained that I was going in this time not because I was sick or needed special care but simply so I could have the best possible supervision, help, and rest while I was going through this important transition.

My insurance completely covered my stay (except the cable TV!), so if money is your concern, talk to your insurance company. If your doctor deems this option to be a medical necessity, insurance should pay for your stay. I understand that in recent years, it takes more of a fight on the doctor's and patient's parts to insure a fully covered hospital stay.

Remember, it takes some time to determine what your basal rates should be, and your first calculations may be off. Until you get your basal rates right, you may experience either hypo- or hyperglycemia. Again, these conditions are treated in different ways when you're on the pump—you can increase or decrease your basal rates and add additional insulin if you need to. Being in this hospital while you are learning to handle these situations allows you optimal safety and peace of mind.

But what do they do in a hospital that I can't do at home?

For one thing, it is critical that you wake up during the night every few hours during those first few days in order to set your nighttime basal rates. Being in the hospital insures that you will be woken, your blood sugar will be checked, and any adjustments that are necessary will be made. Nighttime can be the greatest time of anxiety for new pumpers, but being in the hospital during your first few pumping days is a great antidote to this fear.

If you have a friend or family member who can make a commitment to be there for you during those first nights of pumping, you may be just fine at home. This support person needs to make sure that you wake up and test your blood sugar according to your doctor's orders. Again, before your basal rates are properly set, it could be dangerous to sleep through the entire night. Incorrect basal rates could lead to either hypo- or hyperglycemia. If you are transitioning to the pump at home, make sure that you are clear with your doctor about when you need to call him to check in. If you wake up at 3 A.M. with a blood sugar of 350 mg/dL, will you know what to do? Can you call him at home?

Pumper Gary Russell was shocked to discover how widely your blood sugars can range without long-acting insulin. "The highs are higher and the lows are lower," he warns. That means that you need to learn how to lower or bring up your blood sugar immediately. Judy Swenson recalls how surprised she was by how much bolus insulin she needed to take in order to bring a high blood sugar down to the normal range when she first went on the pump. "My first few days, I would go up to three or four hundred and take what bolus I thought would bring it down. An hour would go by, and no change! Finally I called my doctor, and he yelled at me. 'Why did you wait to call me?' he said. I figured I knew how diabetes works . . . but I really didn't know how to adjust my pump," she explains. Judy also learned an important trick about bringing down her blood sugar during those days: No matter how much she bolused insulin, she couldn't bring down her blood sugars if she wasn't drinking substantial amounts of water. Her body was dehydrated when her sugars were high and couldn't process the insulin she bolused efficiently. None of this information is meant to scare or intimidate you. But you should know that whether you are in the hospital or not, during those first few days of pumping, you need to be in constant touch with your health care provider, test your sugars regularly, and make sure that you wake up every few hours during the night. From the first moment that you go on the pump, you need to react instantaneously. Because you don't have long-acting insulin as a "back-up" in your system, it is dangerous to let high blood sugars go untreated. Likewise, if you see that your blood sugars keep falling, it is necessary to lower your basal rates immediately.

I have so many responsibilities right now, and if I wait until I can take a few days off work, I'll never get started on the pump! Can't I get adjusted while I continue my life?

Ultimately, that decision is up to you. During the first few days of my pumping, I had gotten coverage for my teaching jobs and had told my professors I wouldn't be in class (I was going full-time for my master's degree). Miraculously, the world continued just fine without me being there! We all imagine ourselves to be at the center of the universe and many people with diabetes whom I've met happen to be overachieving, type-A perfectionists. In my opinion, giving yourself a little vacation from your normal responsibilities will help to insure a successful transition into your pump therapy. Besides, I ended up having a great time in the hospital! While I was getting my basal rates set, friends came by to visit. My brother came up to Philadelphia from Washington, D.C. to hang out. I watched TV and read magazines. Frankly, those were two and a half of the most relaxing days I can remember!

Liessa Demba got started on pump therapy in a very different way. "I knew there was never going to be a good time to take off work and I just had to do it now," she recalls. Liessa got hooked up to her pump in the morning and went back to her office a few hours later. She was in constant touch with her diabetes educator, who helped her set her basal rates. It took some time to really find the right rates, but she feels that she got settled into her new routine pretty quickly and easily, while maintaining all of her other life responsibilities at the same time. Liessa had thoroughly educated herself about pump therapy before getting connected, and felt ready to act—with her educator's support—if her blood sugars were running too high or too low. Liessa was fine juggling the newness of the pump with her work responsibilities, and reports a smooth transition.

I really hate hospitals and it will make me feel weird not being at home. What can I do to make my transition successful at home?

"I went into the hospital for two nights when I got started on my pump," recalls Carys Price. "I thought, 'What am I doing here?' The bed was so stiff! It was fine to be there, but didn't feel totally necessary to me."

Again, if going into the hospital is not an option or desire for you, you'll do just fine as long as you make some special preparations. First of all, make sure that you have someone to stay with you at night who will be reliable in helping you get up every two hours to check your blood sugar. Make sure you can reach your doctor by telephone at any hour of the day or night. Try to take time off from work or family responsibilities for a few days. You will need to focus your attention on learning the ins and outs of the pump. Your blood sugars may fluctuate greatly as you try to find your correct basal rates and learn to bolus properly. While these initial days can be trying, they are definitely worth it. As you start to master pump therapy, you will gain an incredible new sense of ease and control.

TEN WAYS
to Prepare for Your
Pump Transition

1. Talk to your doctor or educator about the possibility of being admitted to the hospital. Talk about the advantages and disadvantages of this decision.

2. Mark out some time on your calendar and decide which responsibilities you can release for your first week of pumping. Find someone else to take your day in car pool, cancel non-urgent meetings, etc.

3. Discuss taking a few days off from work. If this is not an option for you, make sure that you can spend time on the phone with your doctor or educator while you're on the job.

4. Find a family member or friend who will be your "nighttime buddy" and insure that you wake up to test your sugars.

5. Call your doctor or educator immediately when sugars are too high or low.

6. Be patient—it takes everyone some time to find the correct basal rates and learn to bolus properly.

7. Keep great records—record everything you eat, all activity, etc. These factors will all affect your basal rates.

8. Take time to relax when you can—you are making a major life transition.

9. Speak with other pumpers or put questions out on the pumpers' list serve.

10. If you have a technical question, call the pump company's 800 number immediately.

PART FOUR

Happily Pumping Ever After . . .

YOU HAVE MADE a great decision—you're hooked up to your pump and have your basal rates set. So why do you feel so . . . overwhelmed? Remember, successful insulin pumping is a process, and it takes most pumpers an average of three to six months to feel completely comfortable with pump therapy.

Even then, pump therapy requires constant commitment and discipline. As Kim Seeley explained, the pump is just a machine—and it is you, the pump user, who has to "think like a pancreas" and use the pump most effectively.

As you become adjusted to pump therapy, some minor issues may arise. You may have an occasional problem with an insertion site, or have trouble getting rid of air bubbles in your insulin cartridges. In this section of the book I address these concerns and offer tips to help resolve them.

For many longtime veterans of diabetes, keeping up the motivation needed for ongoing, optimal diabetes care can be difficult, and even with the pump, you may find yourself dealing with issues of motivation and, at times, even depression. You will hear from other pumpers about ways they overcome these difficulties.

Despite any minor setbacks, feel confident that you have made the choice to use the very best technology out there to work with your diabetes and that this commitment speaks volumes about the respect you give to your own life.

SIXTEEN

The First Few Weeks

YOU'VE MADE IT through the first few days. You're feeling more confident and are ready to get back into the swing of your life. But still—the pump feels so new. You can't remember everything in your manual . . . the beeps are driving you crazy . . . what to do?

Again, the analogy that comes to my mind is that of bringing home a new baby. You are delighted with happiness and excitement at your new arrival—but it does not make it any easier when your baby cries with colic or won't breastfeed. Your pump—wonderful as it is—takes some time to get used to, and like a new parent trying to understand her baby's cries, it will take you some time to fully understand all of the pump's features.

Matthew Lore recalls his initial reactions to pump therapy: "After a first week of hating it, or at least feeling like my blood glucose levels were never going to stabilize, and that it was just so much technology to do what I'd been doing just fine, it all just clicked, and I started to get it, and I totally, totally fell for it." If you are like Matthew, and it clicks in your first week, you are off to a great start.

For others, it can be a good month, or even more, until you reach that "click" moment when everything falls into balance.

Yerachmiel Altman, who had lost much of his vision before starting pump therapy, recalls feeling so much healthier, almost initially. He had family members who helped him do the "technical" stuff like changing infusion sites, and within months of being on the pump, vision returned in one of his eyes. "The little problems didn't matter to me," he says. "Getting my health back to normal did."

Things are not "clicking" with me and the pump, and I don't feel better at all. How long should I wait it out before I chuck the whole thing and go back to injections?

One of the greatest aspects of pump therapy is that you are not making a permanent commitment; the pump is not implanted in your body. If you really feel that it is not the best thing for you, there is no problem with disconnecting and going back to multiple injection therapy. Remember, Sonia Seifert decided to quit pump therapy after two years of pumping! (Only to return to it, on her own terms, a few months later.)

The rule of thumb among pump users is that you should give pump therapy at least three to six months before making a decision to give up on it. "My first four or five months, I absolutely hated the thing," Kim Seeley explains. "It seemed like some alarm was always going off, the tubing was clogged, or something was going wrong! But I stuck with it, and learned that these problems could easily be solved." What resolve made Kim stick with it? Why was it worth it to her to persevere through annoying alarms? "It was the first time in my life that I could adjust my insulin for the changes that happen around my menstrual cycle. I could exercise with better blood sugar control. I could sleep late and eat what I wanted . . . when you compare the so-called 'problems' with all of that, they aren't really a big deal," she says.

Dave Cohen really liked the convenience of his new pump but hated the fact that he had to test his blood sugar much more than before to keep his blood sugars in good control. "It was like, if I didn't test, my sugars could go really high and I wouldn't know it. I never had so many high when I was on Ultralente insulin. I couldn't figure out why my doctor said the pump was better for control," he explained. What Dave needed in order to make his pump transition smoother was more help with carbohydrate counting, and more information about how to take correction boluses of insulin. Once he got those pieces, things started to "click" for him.

The reality is that everyone needs different amounts of support and education on the many pieces that make insulin pump therapy work as a successful treatment system. If one area of pumping is getting you down when you first start, don't be ashamed or embarrassed to ask your medical care team for more help. As with all things in life, there is a very long learning curve for pump therapy.

It's been over a month now that I've been on the pump and I feel like I'm annoying my doctor with all of my questions! But every day I think of something new to ask.

When your health is at stake, you can never ask too many questions. Once you've been on the pump for a few weeks, new questions will continue to arise and there's nothing wrong with seeking the answers that you need.

First of all, never hesitate to call the pump manufacturers directly. Technical service reps at the toll-free lines are available for you night or day. I called during those first weeks with many, many questions— mainly because I wanted reassurance. Their staffers know that new pumpers have many questions and they are always ready to hear from you.

I had one evening—around midnight—when I changed my pump batteries, and still the alarm that signals a low battery kept coming on. I was exhausted and convinced that I was doing something wrong. The more times I changed the batteries, the more frequent the alarm would ring. An hour later, I finally called for technical assistance and found out that I had a batch of defective batteries. The rep had me try each battery in my ten-pack until we found two that were okay. The next day they FedExed me more batteries. Had I not made that phone call, I never would have known that batteries could be defective (so simple, looking back!) and I would have plagued myself for hours, risking a high blood sugar all the while.

Keep your pump manuals with you at all times during those first weeks so that you won't feel pressured to remember everything about the pump at once. It is a lot of information to take in. You'll learn it all in time. If you have your manual close by when you're at work, on the train, or even out to dinner, you'll have a better idea of what to do in case of a problem. Also, refresh yourself by watching the videos about pumping that your pump company gave you with your start-up kit; sometimes, the more you watch, the more it will all click!

Use the support people you've found to talk about what you're going through. Even after you've made the decision to go on the pump, you may experience anxiety as you get started. This is normal and it will pass. Talking to fellow pumpers will make all the difference. Initially, I thought I was the only person in the world who struggled with getting big air bubbles out of my tubing! I couldn't tell the difference between a slight mark in the tube and a real bubble that was stopping my insulin from getting through. An experienced pumper taught me a great trick: Hold your tubing up against a dark background, like a navy pillowcase or sweater. It's much easier to recognize air bubbles that way, and priming the tubing will move them right through. Again, an experienced pumper will gladly answer those unanticipated questions that will surely come up for you. We understand; we've been there.

TEN WAYS

TO "COPE" DURING YOUR
FIRST FEW WEEKS PUMPING

1. Remember that most people go through a period of adjustment that can take as little as a week or as long as a year.

2. Make a commitment to stick with pump therapy for at least six months before you decide to change your diabetes treatment.

3. When you have medical questions, call your doctor or diabetes educator. That's what they are there for!

4. Call your pump's 800 number when you have any technical support questions—day or night.

5. Keep your pump instruction manual with you wherever you go.

6. Make sure to have *all* of your diabetes care supplies with you at all times.

7. Reach out to other pump users for support and guidance.

8. Let family, friends, and loved ones know that you are going through a major transition, in case you don't quite seem like "yourself."

9. Keep reading and learning about pump therapy.

10. Go back for more education in any trouble spots. If you need nutritional counseling, now is the ideal time to get it.

SEVENTEEN

Weight Management and the Pump: Watching Those Pounds

MANY PEOPLE GAIN a few—up to five—pounds when they first go on pump therapy. There, I've said it! It is actually a good thing: Your body is adjusting to this healthy change and processing insulin much more normally. You will level off within a few months and will not continue to gain weight without cause.

That is, unless you're like some of us . . . who just couldn't resist eating absolutely everything in sight when we started pumping! You see, you can figure out how much insulin to bolus to cover ice cream, cakes, cookies . . . food you may have very well been told to avoid in the past. I went through a bit of a splurge when I first started pumping. I had been really good since I was ten years old, avoiding sweets in day-to-day life to keep my blood sugars in tight control. With the pump, I could now try dessert and keep my sugars okay. I started experimenting . . . Ben & Jerry's needs this much bolus; Sara Lee takes a few units more . . . hey, this pump thing is really fun! I honestly wasn't thinking about my weight until I started noticing my clothes getting a little snug . . . and three months after starting the pump, the scale at the doctor's office said I'd put on twelve pounds!

Yikes! So embarrassing to look back on now. That news was my wake-up call.

Do I have to stay on a "diabetic" diet when I'm on the pump?

Although you could eat whatever you want and maintain good blood sugar control, the pump should not be an excuse to avoid good nutrition. In my experience, I realized that excessive sweets aren't healthy for anyone, whether you have or don't have diabetes. I increased my workouts, ate more salads instead of sweets, and dropped most of the excess weight pretty easily. I now incorporate low-fat ice cream or frozen yogurt into my meal plan for the week . . . but I eat it moderately, as part of a very balanced diet . . . not as my main course! Be conscious of this trap when you start pumping . . . nutritional common sense still prevails. If you find yourself having a hard time resisting junk-food temptations, seek help from a nutritionist.

Kathy Kochan, whose cookbooks offer healthy recipes for everyone—with or without diabetes—believes strongly in nutrition as one of the main components for people with diabetes to feel their best—along with insulin and exercise. She creates recipes that everyone enjoys, for low-carbohydrate, healthy eating. "It's all about balance,"

Kathy explains. "I love to eat cookies. If I decide to eat a cookie for lunch, I won't eat bread." Notice she says "a cookie," not "a box of cookies." The pump can be a great tool in creating a healthier diet—you will be able to discern exactly how specific foods affect your blood sugar and work with that information more effectively.

There really is no longer a "diabetic diet" as in years gone by. Today nutritionists recommend that people with diabetes follow nutrition guidelines that are healthy for the general population: eating high-fiber foods, low-glycemic carbohydrates, with lean proteins, some fat, and plenty of fruits and vegetables.

Sure, you can still indulge in the occasional dessert or eat some sweet foods that you never did before—but do so moderately, with an eye toward nutritional balance.

Yerachmiel Altman credits years on the Pritikin diet plan, along with pump therapy, for contributing to his excellent health despite having diabetes since age two. "Pritikin, a diet plan full of vegetables and fiber, is extremely compatible with pump therapy," he explains. Good nutrition practices can take time to incorporate, but having the opportunity to better control your blood sugars can be a great motivator in improving every aspect of your health, which a balanced diet ensures.

I was about thirty pounds overweight when I started on my pump and I really want to get the weight off. How do I do it?

If only there were a magical answer! As any of us who have struggled with weight issues know, cutting calories and increasing exercise is the only surefire way to safely lose those pounds.

When you decide to lose weight and you're on the pump, consult with your doctor about how to do so safely. When you lose weight, you will need to adjust your basal rates. If you are exercising more and eating less, you will need to lower your basal rates to avoid hypoglycemia. If you are eating fewer calories, you will also be taking less bolus insulin.

Many, many pump users report that weight loss is easier than ever. Again—no more eating to "feed" your insulin. If you want to skip a meal or snack, you can. If you want to eat significantly fewer calories, you can. You will be able to exercise without getting low blood sugar. All of these factors make the pump a great tool for people with diabetes to use in a successful weight-loss program.

TEN FACTORS

1. Many people put on a couple of pounds during their first few months of pumping. Not to worry—it's a normal part of your body adjusting to using insulin more efficiently.

2. If you gain over five pounds, talk to your doctor or nutritionist about weight-management strategies.

3. Eat sweets and other treats in moderation. Just because you can bolus for them doesn't mean that they're calorie free or good for you!

4. Keep good records to discern how certain foods affect your blood sugar. If you need to take a very high bolus of insulin to cover a certain food, you may want to consider eliminating that food item from your diet.

5. Read up on good nutrition—ask your doctor or nutritionist for recommendations.

6. Make exercise a part of your life—explore new forms of exercise that interest you.

7. Log on to the Diabetes Exercise and Sports Association Web site to place questions about exercise and diabetes (www.diabetes-exercise.org).

8. Seek support or join a weight-management group to explore emotional connections to eating and weight-related issues.

9. Talk to your doctor about healthy ways to lose weight. Cut basal rates and boluses as needed.

10. Remember that diabetes management involves many aspects—insulin dosaging, diet, exercise . . . and, of course, staying emotionally healthy.

EIGHTEEN

Troubleshooting the Bumps in the Road

I WISH I could tell you that once you master the basics of pumping, you will never have any glitches with pump therapy. Realistically, this ideal scenario will not be the case. But, however, the good news is that the problems you'll encounter should be relatively minor ones . . . and with experience in how to deal with them, they'll be little "bumps in the road" of your smooth path to pumping with ease.

So far, so good. I've been pumping for six months and haven't had any problems. What kind of thing should I be looking out for?

Many pumpers will go along for some time without any problems at all. However, you should be aware of what to look out for—so that you can prevent these problems if possible and know how to deal with them should they arise.

The most common pump problems have to do with the insertion site, and we'll break them down, one by one. Issues include infections, sweating, bleeding, and allergic reactions.

Taking good care of your insertion site is key to pump therapy success. Insertion sites need to be changed every forty-eight hours for metal needles and every forty-eight to seventy-two hours for Teflon cannula sets (the preferred infusion site set). Individuals may vary among how long they can go before changing an infusion set. If a set is not changed in a timely fashion, then insulin can't be absorbed properly under the skin, causing high blood sugar.

The best way to ensure an infection-free infusion site is to keep your skin nice and clean when changing sites. Most pumpers like to put in a clean site right when they get out of a shower. You can also clean your skin with alcohol, an antiseptic pad, or Purell (a skin disinfectant) to further prevent any chance of infection. Parents should be aware that some children are especially sensitive to alcohol-based products; test your child's skin sensitivity before using a product to prep for an infusion site.

If you see any swelling or redness at your site, or feel discomfort or pressure when you touch it, change your infusion site immediately. If your skin stays red or swollen or is painful to the touch, you may have an infection and need to call your doctor immediately.

I find it uncomfortable to change my infusion set and really dread doing so. Is there any way to make the insertion more comfortable?

People vary widely in their tolerance for discomfort. Most pumpers, veteran needle-givers, have no problem with insertion sets, while other people react strongly to them. First of all, it is recommended that you speak with your pump company about their recommendation for their most "comfortable" set available. Second, you may want to explore whether you are choosing the most ideal insertion site on your body. Most pumpers use the abdomen (staying two inches away from the navel) but many others prefer the hip, thigh, or even upper arm. The rule goes that if you can "pinch an inch," you can insert there. Some people may experience discomfort inserting in their abdomen if they have virtually no inch of fat there, and will feel much better using a hip or thigh.

Some simple techniques that can ease the discomfort of changing your insertion site include:

- Applying ice or an ice pack to your skin for several minutes before inserting.
- Applying EMLA (a prescription cream that numbs skin) an hour before inserting the infusion set.
- Using an insertion device for your infusion set, which can decrease pain and help make certain the set is inserted properly.
- Making sure that you are rotating sites effectively, staying at least an inch away from the previous site.

Besides discomfort, you want to make sure to rotate your insertion sites so that you don't build up lumpy, fibrous tissue. Taking that extra minute to find a good site will help your skin stay healthy in the long run.

KID'S CORNER

Finding the Best Site

FINDING A good infusion site for children, who have smaller body mass than adults, can be a challenge. The "pinch an inch" rule may not work here; however, many parents have had success with the "if it bends, don't insert" rule. You may need to rotate from the abdomen to the buttocks or hips and use a different style of infusion set, depending where you insert.

It is critical to test prior to changing a site and then to test again, two hours later. If your child's blood sugar is unexplainably high, you probably have a bad sight and need to change it immediately.

I tend to sweat a lot and my infusion set shifts out of place. What can I do?

Another common, but fortunately easy to solve problem! As I discussed in the exercise chapter, excessive sweating can cause major problems should an infusion site become loose and fall out. If you tend to perspire a great deal, you can apply an antiperspirant (followed by a rub with an antiseptic pad) onto your skin before inserting your infusion set. You can also cover the tabs of your insertion site with extra adhesive tape to keep the set in place. As long as you keep an extra eye on your set, all should go well. If you have an unexplained high blood sugar reading, check your site immediately. It may have come loose, preventing your insulin from being absorbed.

I had an episode in which blood squirted out when I removed my infusion site. How can I prevent this kind of thing from happening again?

"It was great," Dave Cohen remembers. "Just like an episode of *E.R.* I was changing my site and the next thing I knew, blood was gushing out like crazy!" Dave remembers this one-time incident as one of his more exciting events with the pump, but if you're like many of us who aren't crazy about gushing blood, you'll want to know how to prevent such an episode.

Occasionally, a blood vessel near the surface of the skin can get nicked when the needle of an infusion site enters the skin. Often when this happens, you will feel a slight discomfort and should take your infusion site out. If you don't feel that discomfort, you may see a red area forming at the infusion site. Carefully and slowly remove your infusion set, and have a towel ready to put pressure on the area of affected skin to stop the bleeding.

Bleeding should stop within a few minutes and you can apply a warm compress to the affected area. Be sure to clean the skin with alcohol and cover with a Band-Aid. Watch for any signs of infection near the area, and call your doctor immediately if you think you may have an infection and/or if your blood sugars stay high for no reason.

"In all of my two and a half years of pumping, I started bleeding only one time when I changed my infusion set," says Cara Jennings. "It was not fun, but it stopped pretty quickly. I was more shocked than anything, because no one had ever told me that that could happen. I asked my doctor about it and she just sort of said, 'Oh, yeah, it could happen.' I think if it happened again, I would stay more calm about the whole thing."

As Cara points out, knowledge is the key to being prepared and dealing with these occasional pump inconveniences.

My skin is red and bumpy when I change my site. What's going on? What can I do?

When Yerachmiel Altman first started pumping, steel needles were the only possible way to insert an infusion site into the skin. He developed an allergic reaction to the metal, waking up one day with an infection the size of a golf ball under his skin. "There were no Teflon infusion sets available then, so my doctor had me go to a pharmacy and get Teflon IV needles and adhesive tape. That's how I got my infusion sites in for years, until they started producing the Teflon sets," he remembers. Such allergies, while not common, do occur from time to time.

More difficult to cope with is an allergic reaction to adhesive tape. Some pumpers have found that using extra rubbing alcohol and an antibiotic cream can lessen the reaction. There are now nonallergenic adhesive products on the market. There is the rare person who has stopped pumping insulin because of a severe adhesive tape allergy.

TEN WAYS

TO TROUBLESHOOT INFUSION SET PROBLEMS

1. Change your site regularly—every two to three days, depending on your set.

2. Find the best place on your body to insert your infusion set.

3. Look regularly for any sign of infection—change your infusion site immediately if you have discomfort, your skin is red or swollen, or your blood sugar is unexplainably high.

4. If you think you may have an infection, call your doctor immediately.

5. If you are an "excessive" sweater, take precautions to keep your infusion site in place.

6. A red area at the site may mean you've nicked a blood vessel; change infusion site slowly and have a towel ready to stop any bleeding that may occur.

7. Be sure to rotate at least one inch away from your previous site.

8. You may want to show a friend or family member how to change your infusion site in the event that you are ill and need help doing the change.

9. If you notice consistent red or bumpy patches of skin, see your doctor right away.

10. Always clean your skin (and hands!) before changing infusion sites.

NINETEEN

Your Emotional Health

ANYONE DEALING WITH a chronic health issue faces a variety of emotional challenges. Diabetes certainly presents a great many challenges to cope with and worry about, and studies indicate that a large number of people with diabetes deal with chronic or episodal bouts of depression. In my opinion, the connection between diabetes and depression is one of the great, neglected causes of our times.

It's a "chicken-and-egg" question: What comes first, the diabetes or the depression? Are people with a greater tendency toward depression more vulnerable to diabetes, or vice versa? Certainly living with ongoing states of high blood sugar saps one's energy and life force, leading to feelings of loss and hopelessness. And being stuck in a depressed state can make a person lack all motivation to take care of him- or herself. How much effort can a severely depressed person put into maintaining good blood sugar control? How does a bleak world view affect personal diabetes care?

Yet, how many endocrinologists raise the issue of depression during their visits with their patients? And how many patients are comfortable confiding in their physicians that their depression is what's been impairing them from taking better care of their health?

"No one touches the emotional side of living with diabetes," Yerachmiel Altman states. "My diabetes was making me so depressed, so my wife finally came with me to the doctor and said, 'Do something to help him!' You see, I wasn't taking great care of myself then, but when I got my diabetes under control again, my depression went away." Yerachmiel, who had been on the early insulin pump, had thought he knew everything there was to know about managing diabetes. But when his doctor suggested that he go back and take some refresher courses, he was willing to try it. He took some diabetes education classes in carbohydrate counting and pump management, and was able to get his blood sugars under much better control through his newfound knowledge. And the bonus: With better blood sugar control came a relief from his depression!

KIDS'S CORNER

Diabetes: A Family Illness

EMOTIONAL ISSUES connected to diabetes do not only affect the individual with diabetes. Often in families in which one child has diabetes, his or her sibling can feel left out, jealous, and alienated by the "attention" that the child with diabetes receives. Though he or she may rationally know that diabetes doesn't seem like much fun, it is still hard to feel like one can compete for a parent's attention against such an ever-pervasive distraction.

Parents should look for ways to give all siblings their fair share of attention, and to allow the child without diabetes to express his or her feelings about the illness. Sometime just including siblings in the "realities" of diabetes—such as counting carbs—can help to normalize it for everyone.

Many people on pump therapy report a kind of "lift" in spirit and outlook that goes along with their A1cs becoming lower. "I never thought of myself as being a 'depressed' person," says Judy Swenson.

"But I guess I always felt a little hopeless about my diabetes. And I never realized, until I started pumping insulin, how generally sluggish and slow I felt. My blood sugars used to bounce around everywhere, and I didn't think to myself that that could be affecting my moods and my energy."

The good news is that getting blood sugars under control can be a great help in aiding depression, and the new sense of control over your body and health can help to create a more positive outlook on life. The pump is certainly not a "cure" for depression, but good blood sugar control may play a role in helping to stabilize your moods.

TEEN TIPS

Signs of Depression

MOOD SWINGS are a normal part of the teenage years, right? Yes and no. While most teenagers experience heightened emotions at one point or another, teens facing serious, ongoing depressed states of mind need intervention and help. If your teenager has sudden shifts in sleep patterns (insomnia or sleeping all the time), eating (bingeing or starving), social life (changing friends, staying at home instead of going to after-school activities, etc.) or is having problems at school, it may be time for an evaluation.

In addition to depression, eating disorders like anorexia and bulimia can wreak havoc on a teen's life. For teenagers with diabetes, eating disorders can be truly life-threatening and require immediate medical care.

Since I've started pump therapy, I feel more depressed. I thought this was supposed to make me feel better! What's going on?

"I think, in a certain way, I felt a bit more depressed after I'd been on the pump," Cara Jennings says. "Because before that, when things were wrong in my life or I had crazy moods, I'd say, 'Oh, it's my blood sugar making me nuts!' But when I got my sugars under such good control, it was like . . . okay, something else is causing my mood swings. What's going on?" Once you deal with feelings around your diabetes, other emotional issues may have room to surface. Hopefully, your commitment to getting your diabetes in optimal control will help you face other life issues that may be affecting your health, including issues of emotional well-being. Once you're acclimated to the pump, it might be the ideal time to start therapy or join a support group. It's easy to get caught in the trap of "blaming" our diabetes for all that isn't happy or right in our lives. Taking control of one's diabetes opens room in our emotional life to take charge of other issues and lose the "victim" mentality once and for all!

WORD TO THE WISE

Pumps and the Mentally Ill

PEOPLE WHO suffer from mental illness, such as schizophrenia or other psychotic disorders, are not recommended as candidates for pump therapy. Unfortunately, the parameters of their illness may prohibit them from being able to attend to the responsibilities connected with pump therapy.

I've never had a problem with depression, but have major trouble coping with stress. Even pump therapy hasn't helped me with that. HELP!!!

Many people forget that besides feeling unpleasant, "stress" causes a physiological reaction in our bodies. Your body goes into "fight or flight" mode and releases stress hormones into your blood. Stress hormones actually release stored up glucose or fat into your blood, and if your body does not have enough insulin in its system, you know what will occur: high blood sugar. If you are on pump therapy, your normal basal rates cannot provide enough insulin for a whopping bout of stress. To make matters more complicated, some people seem to react to stress hormones in the opposite way, and severe stress can lead to low blood sugar levels.

"I think people don't realize how destructive stress can be," reports Carys Price. "When I deal with work stress, my blood sugars can run really, really high. If I don't tune in to what's going on, I'm in trouble." Fortunately, Carys is aware of her body's reaction to stress and also knows what her personal stress triggers are.

Stress doesn't always have to be a bad thing—we can release adrenaline when we're happy or excited, but it still affects our blood sugar. When I first started on pump therapy, I was shocked at how much my blood sugars would rise after a two-hour teaching session. I could go in at 100, and leave at 275! I didn't consider myself "stressed" while I taught, but always exerted a tremendous amount of energy. Feeding off my students' energy really got my adrenaline going, which further fueled the cycle. I learned that I had to test my blood sugar an hour into teaching, take a bolus as needed, keep drinking water, and remember to slow down and breathe deeply even when I was passionate about a point I was making!

If you are in a job or life situation that is causing you chronic stress, it may be having an impact on your blood sugar that you are not aware of. Try to find ways to counter the stress—explore deep breathing and meditation techniques, yoga, visualization, exercise, massage, or psychotherapy. If you still cannot stop the stress, it is time to consider making a life change that will bring you greater peace of mind. Your emotional health and physical health are connected, and constantly feeding off each other. Even a switch to pump therapy can't insure good blood sugar control unless you find some emotional balance.

TEN THINGS

TO KNOW ABOUT DIABETES
AND EMOTIONAL HEALTH

1. A large number of people living with diabetes also deal with depression.

2. It is important to acknowledge your depression with your doctor, difficult as it may be to talk about.

3. High blood sugar has an effect on emotional well-being—making one sluggish and low in energy.

4. Insulin pump therapy can help you gain normal blood sugar control, bringing moods to a more even keel.

5. Emotional issues—and depression—may still arise when you're on pump therapy. Always seek help for such problems.

6. A diabetes support group can help make you feel less isolated in dealing with issues about diabetes.

7. Stress also plays a role in elevating blood glucose.

8. "Good stress"—like excitement—can still raise blood glucose.

9. Strategies for dealing with stress include deep breathing and meditation techniques, yoga, visualization, exercise, massage, and psychotherapy.

10. Remember—your physical and emotional well-being are connected, and both parts of your health need attention and care.

TWENTY

Staying Motivated

ONE EMOTIONAL/PHYSICAL health issue that deserves a chapter of its own is motivation. People with diabetes need an enormous reserve of this sometimes elusive quality. For people on insulin pump therapy, motivation is a key component to successful pumping. Without the will to constantly check blood sugars, adjust basal rates, take proper boluses, as well as exercise, count carbs, change infusion sites, etc., people on pump therapy can find that their blood sugars aren't much better controlled than they were before they went on the pump. Pump therapy requires moment-by-moment attention; without long-acting insulin in your system, any lapse in your care could lead to an extremely high or low blood sugar.

I've been on the pump for two and a half years, and had excellent A1cs during my first two years. The last six months have been off. I just don't have the drive to check my sugars as much as I used to. What's going on?

"At first when I got my pump, I was so anal and excited about the whole thing," Kim Seeley says. "Then it got kind of old. The whole routine. It gets hard to stay motivated at times." Kim's feelings are echoed by many, many pump users. It is probably a totally unrealistic goal to imagine that since you're on pump therapy, you will always strive to maintain your best control ever. It is a perfectionists' view of living with diabetes that few of us can live up to. Which doesn't mean that anyone's encouraging you to slack off! It just means that if you have a day or a week or a month in which your blood sugars aren't perfect, don't beat yourself up and make it worse! "I always wished I could just take a vacation from my diabetes every once in a while," says Cara Jennings. "Like if I could take a week off and not deal, I know I'd do so much better than I was doing before."

Ahhh—to dream of such a day! For now it seems that the best we can do is to try to stay aware of any patterns of lack of motivation that may arise, and find a new strategy to get us excited about our diabetes care again.

While we can't take a "vacation" from our diabetes, we can find people to vent our frustrations with. We can let a friend or loved one know when we're down, and seek a bit of encouragement. Sometimes finding a new passion or interest in life can give us the lift we need—and remind us that it's worth fighting the good fight, because life has so many wonderful experiences to offer. And sometimes we just need to have an all-out "pity" day . . . and if we don't check our sugars as often as we should, or if we eat junk food that's really not good for us, so be it. Our diabetes won't go away, but it's only human to acknowledge that we can't be perfect all the time.

KIDS' CORNER

A Break for Mom and Dad

IF PARENTS are fortunate enough to have a set of grandparents or other close relatives or friends who are willing to become fully educated about pump therapy, encourage them to do so. You can train Grandma or Grandpa to do all the things you normally do: check blood sugars, adjust for boluses, change insulin cartridges, etc. The training may take some time, just as it did for you. If your friend or relative wants to keep your child for an afternoon (or even a weekend), let them try it. As long as they are educated and have experience working with your child's pump, and you are reachable at all times by phone, then you can let them take over the primary responsibility for a short time.

Many parents who take such a break from "thinking like their child's pancreas" report that they are more patient and relaxed when their son or daughter comes home.

I feel overwhelmed by how much effort I need to put into my diabetes care. I need to lose weight, get into a fitness routine, check my blood sugars more frequently. It just all shuts me down.

There are so many different aspects to balancing one's health, and with diabetes present, the challenges are that much more present and urgent. Talk to your doctor or educator about setting short-term goals and tackling one issue at a time. Amazingly, working on one area of your health care may naturally lead you to fix another. For example, if you start by focusing on an exercise plan, you may start to feel better in general and start wanting to eat a more nutritionally-balanced diet. Make short-term goals clear, specific, and manageable to achieve. Achieving optimal diabetes care is a process, and even once we've "gotten" it, we are going to hit times when we get stuck all over again.

Ernie and Liessa Demba
—Father and Daughter Speak Out on Successful Pumping

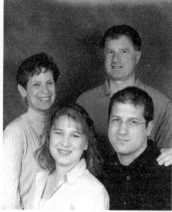

The Demba family

FOR BOTH Ernie and Liessa Demba, a desire to stay as healthy as possible, to not miss out on any daily activities, and to simply feel as good as possible motivates their diabetes care routine. Ernie chose pump therapy twenty years ago, when despite the mechanical and electrical problems, he found that pump therapy allowed him the greatest lifestyle flexibility and the best way to tighten blood sugar control. Liessa, in turn, grew up in a family in which both diabetes and the insulin pump were both "normal" (her brother also has type 1 diabetes) parts of life, allowing her to easily accept her chronic illness.

Ernie reflects that when he needed motivation in the early days, he thought of his young children and how he wanted to live a healthy life to be around for them. Liessa, who hopes to start a family soon, also thinks about the implications of being a mother when she needs an extra dose of diabetes motivation.

While Ernie acknowledges that it's not always easy for a parent with diabetes to step back and watch as his kids come to their own terms with figuring out how important tight blood sugar control is, he also realizes that having more than one person with diabetes in a family has the benefit of creating a built-in support system. Liessa, now an adult, realizes how much work it took on both her father's and mother's parts to raise her and her brother in such a way that diabetes was just a part of life. "What a blessing," she says.

Both Ernie and Liessa credit pump therapy with allowing them to live busy, hectic, healthy lives. As Liessa puts it, "Pump therapy is my ticket to success."

TEN WAYS

TO DEAL WITH THE
MOTIVATION ISSUE

1. Know that you're not alone—all of us lose our motivation once in a while.

2. Don't panic—motivation is a cyclical thing and will come back to you.

3. Don't keep it to yourself—let friends and family know what you're going through.

4. It could be a good time to talk with other people with diabetes and find out how they get remotivated—check for a support group or meet people on-line.

5. Seek spiritual support or comfort—pastoral professionals may be specially trained to help people dealing with chronic illness.

6. Find something to be excited about in life—try a new hobby, read a new book, take a trip. Sometimes the less that diabetes is a focus, the easier it is to take care of it.

7. Talk to your doctor or diabetes educator—she may offer valuable tips for staying motivated.

8. Set short-term goals. Maybe you can't deal with all aspects of your diabetes at once, but focus on one area that you can work on, such as nutrition.

9. Exercise—even if you have to drag your sorry bones to the gym! Exercise *really* will make you feel better.

10. Laugh! A sense of humor about the daily travails of life with diabetes can go a long way in keeping things in perspective.

TWENTY-ONE

Pump Therapy
and Travel

Since the tragic events of September 11, 2001, Americans have been faced with a wake-up call about airport security. No more breezing through metal detectors and running to catch a plane minutes before takeoff; now we know that we must show up at the airport earlier, go through more thorough security searches, and, at times, experience greater travel delays. For people with diabetes, this situation calls for special preparation.

In the weeks immediately following September 11, I learned about several air travelers with diabetes who were stopped and questioned because of their syringes. Certainly syringes and pump supplies like insertion kits are not everyday items found in most suitcases. Therefore, it is critical to be prepared to calmly and clearly explain what your diabetes supplies are.

The Federal Aviation Administration has implemented the following security guidelines: All insulin vials must come with a pre-printed label coming from a professional pharmacy; in other words, don't discard your insulin box, but save it and bring it if you're traveling by air. The same goes for glucagon kits—keep the packaging with your pharmacy's label. Lancets must be capped and kept with glucose meters. Keeping your prescription or original box for your insulin pump supplies can only help, should you be stopped in a security search.

Please note, the FAA's measures apply only to domestic flights, so if you are planning to travel abroad, be sure to call your airline and find out what their policy is on traveling with diabetes supplies. All of this pre-planning may seem a bit much, but in the long run it's really a small price to pay for better security.

I heard that I need to have a letter from my doctor if I plan to fly. What should it say?

There has been a back-and-forth discussion about the worth of a medical letter of necessity, largely because the airlines have realized how easily such a letter can be forged. Personally, I'm of the "better safe than sorry" school of thought, and keep a letter from my physician on hand anytime that I travel. The letter states:

> To Whom It May Concern:
> Gabrielle Kaplan-Mayer has type 1 (insulin dependent) diabetes. In order to monitor and manage her blood glucose levels, she is required to carry an insulin pump, insulin, a glucose meter and test strips, insulin syringes, and insertion kits, and appropriate prescriptions for her diabetes.

The letter is signed and dated by my doctor. Another very simple thing that can help you in the event of a security problem is to show the security people your medical alert tag (which, of course, you're wearing!). Just having that concrete bit of evidence that you really do have a medical condition works well with security people.

Is my pump going to set off the metal detector?

Probably not. At this juncture, metal detectors are much more likely to catch you if you forget about some loose change in your pocket or are wearing a studded belt. From time to time, pumpers have reported being stopped by a sensitive metal detector.

"I travel quite frequently for my business," Gary Russell explains, "and I'm surprised that I usually pass right through with my pump. The one time I was stopped, I was asked to show a letter from my doctor." In general, most security people will assume that your pump is a beeper, but in the event that you are stopped, you should not be delayed or kept from entering your flight. Clearly and calmly explain what your insulin pump is for.

WORD TO THE WISE

Avoiding the "Big" Search

ANOTHER CONSEQUENCE of September 11, 2001, for airline passengers has been the random selection of passengers for a thorough search of luggage. These searches can happen both at the metal detectors and at the airport gates.

Some pump users prefer to simply take off their pumps and put them in the boxes that are used for keys, etc. to go through the metal detector. This way, the pump at least has no chance of setting off a metal detector and you can thus increase your chances of avoiding a more thorough search.

How do I adjust my basal rates when I'm flying through different time zones?

Adjusting basal rates across different time zones can be a bit of a challenge. For example, my basal rates stay the same from noon until 7 P.M.; from 7 P.M. to midnight they increase by two units. I recently flew from the East Coast to California and had to adjust my basal rates to the time change; while the clock said 5 P.M. when I arrived in California, my body knew I was still at an 8 P.M. "East Coast" basal rate. Depending on the length of your plane ride, you can generally change the clock on your pump at any point during the flight. You may need to take a correction bolus or lower your basal rates as your body starts to adjust. The best way to determine what adjustments you need to make is through frequent blood sugar testing. Check with your doctor for any travel-adjusting tips, especially if you are taking a long international flight.

For pump users who use multiple daily basal rates, long flights through many time zones can be especially challenging. Matthew Lore, who recently took a twenty-one-hour flight from New York to Sydney (including a layover in Los Angeles) tested his blood sugar about a dozen times within that period to make sure that his sugars were staying in a safe range.

Kathy Kochan, a frequent flyer, offers an important tip for pump users: "Never change your infusion set during a flight. First of all, the bathroom is tiny, and secondly, you never know when turbulence will hit!" Kathy is right on—change your infusion site way in advance of boarding your plane.

I'm planning a vacation for next summer, and am going to include a lot of hiking and biking in our plans. What precautions do I need to take?

The greatest part about traveling with the pump is the increased sense of ease and flexibility that is possible. It's no longer a disaster if you miss a meal or if your schedule changes dramatically while on vacation. As long as you keep testing, you can be as flexible in your lifestyle and activity choices as you desire. People who like to take very "active" vacations, filled with biking, mountain climbing, sailing, hiking, etc. are among those who love the pump the most! Talk with your doctor about how you need to adjust your basal rates if you will be doing an extraordinary amount of physical activity. And, of course, pack all of your needed supplies and more, just to be safe. Enjoy the newfound ease of traveling with the pump.

TEN TIPS

FOR TRAVELING
WITH THE PUMP

1. If you are flying, follow the FAA's regulations.

2. Keep a letter from your physician with you—just in case.

3. Pack plenty of supplies—extra stuff is better. Think about how many supplies you need in an average week, then take more.

4. Wear your Medic Alert tag (always!).

5. Keep a "diabetes information card" in your wallet or billfold.

6. If you will be crossing time zones, talk to your physician about how to best adjust your basal rates.

7. Test your blood sugar regularly.

8. Always change an infusion set *before* getting on a plane, train, or into an automobile.

9. Stretch! Whether you're on a long flight, cross-country drive, or riding the Skinny Puppy (Greyhound!), get up or get out during stops and stretch your legs. Keep that circulation flowing!

10. Adjust basal rates as needed for extra activity.

PART FIVE:

Pumping for Everyone! Kids, Teens, Seniors, and Moms-to-Be

IF YOU FALL into one of the special categories listed above, hopefully you've found this book as a whole to be helpful to you. But different life stages can carry specific concerns and challenges regarding pump therapy, so the following chapters offer experiences and advice from folks who've been there.

There are no set barriers about who can or cannot use the insulin pump: The most important factor is the commitment of the pump user (and parents, in the case of children). Remember the story of Yerachmiel Altman, who started pump therapy when he was nearly blind. With the help of family members, he was able to pump successfully. Today many blind people use the pump with equal success—as long as they, and a loved one who can help with some mechanical matters, make the pump therapy commitment.

As always, your medical care team can offer guidance about whether pump therapy is the best treatment choice for you, or someone you love.

TWENTY-TWO

Pumping Kids

INSULIN PUMP THERAPY presents unique challenges for parents of young children: Not only do the parents need to "think like a pancreas" to adjust basal and bolus insulin, they must think that way even when the pancreas is away from them—at school, day care, or staying with a friend! But pump therapy also offers many families a better, more flexible lifestyle choice . . . and gives parents better peace of mind knowing that their child is keeping his or her blood sugars in the normal range.

Research supports the effectiveness of insulin pump therapy in infants and preschool-age children. Dr. Michael Freemark, chief of the division of pediatric endocrinology and diabetes at Duke University, recently released a study stating that "with proper supervision, toddlers and pre-school age children with type 1 diabetes can safely and successfully use an external insulin pump rather than multiple injections to treat their disease." The study involved nine children, between the ages of twenty months and five years, who had developed diabetes between the ages of ten and forty months, and were initially placed on multiple injection therapy (for six months) before moving to pump therapy. The parents of the children received extensive training in the pump as part of the program.

"In young children, food intake and physical activity levels are unpredictable, and it is difficult to administer very low doses of insulin precisely," says Dr. Freemark. "Moreover, the child is often unable to convey symptoms of low blood glucose to parents and caretakers. These factors make diabetic control exceedingly difficult in this age group and increase the risk of severe hypoglycemia."

The study found that hemoglobin A1c levels declined in all patients, from a mean of 9.5 to a 7.9 percent. Also, there was a fivefold decline in the number of episodes of hypoglycemia. Also of note, the frequency of parental contact with medical professionals declined from one contact every 5.9 days to one contact every 46.3 days.

"In conversations, parents stressed their increasing level of comfort with diabetes management, their sense of improvement in quality of life for all family members, and their high levels of satisfaction with pump therapy," Dr. Freemark says.

He does note that pump therapy is not right for all children—families must have strong motivation and commitment to make it work.

One mom who's made that commitment is Jeanine Lore, whose seven-year-old daughter, Abigail, was diagnosed with type 1 diabetes at age five. Abby, niece of Matthew Lore, was initially put on a combination of regular and NPH insulin. "Abby spent a lot of time getting low blood sugars," Jeanine recalls. "We had to feed the insulin rather than feed her when she was hungry, which is extremely difficult with a young child."

Jeanine initially learned about the insulin pump on a diabetes Web site, but when she spoke with Abby's doctor about the possibility of getting her started on pump therapy, he was not altogether enthused about the idea, since Abby had only been diagnosed three months before. Jeanine went on to find other parents whose young children were on the pump, and they gave her a clear picture of what life is like with a kid on the pump. "It's not a pancreas, they explained to me, it's just a tool to help with diabetes management," she explains. Jeanine went on to convince her doctor that this was the right move for her family. Her next challenge was to introduce Abby to the pump.

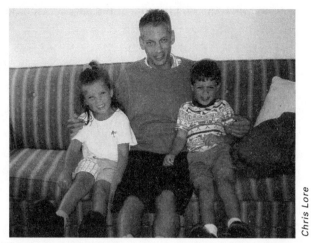

Chris Lore

Abigail and Christopher Lore & their uncle Matthew—Abby & Matthew are both pumpers.

When Jeanine showed Abby a picture of the pump on a Web site, Abby balked. "Her first reaction was that she didn't want to wear it and look different from everybody else. But when I found a picture of Miss America 1999, Nicole Johnson, with her insulin pump, Abby really liked that!" Jeanine recalls.

One advantage Abby quickly figured out was that with the pump, she'd have to be stuck with a needle only every two to three days rather than several times in one day. Abby also insisted that she have a blue insulin pump.

In the beginning, Jeanine remembers a good deal of adjusting. She or Abby's dad, Chris Lore, would wake up at night and check Abby's blood sugar at 10 P.M., 12 A.M., 3 A.M. and 5:30 A.M. It took some time, but soon Abby was able to articulate to her parents when she was feeling high or low blood sugar, which she had not been able to distinguish before.

Even when parents get the pumping routine down at home, they must make sure that caretakers at school know how to work with the pump. Jeanine was fortunate to encounter a school nurse whose own daughter is diabetic, and who was able to understand the mechanics of the pump quite quickly. The nurse has a carbohydrate counting book in her office, and Jeanine writes down the amount of carbs in Abby's lunches. Abby has agreed that she will always eat her sandwich and drink her milk for lunch. Abby goes to the nurse, who supervises her bolus for the sandwich and milk, then Abby heads off to have lunch with her friends. Abby goes back to the nurse after lunch and tells her how much of her actual lunch that she ate: one-half of a yogurt, ten grapes, etc. The nurse determines her bolus, then Abby heads back to class.

Abby wanted to talk with the kids in her class about the pump before she actually wore it to school. Jeanine brought in a book about kids and diabetes and read it to her class, who had plenty of questions. "The kids are pretty infatuated with her leather pump case," Jeanine says, laughing. "Some of the girls in her class really want to be 'diabetic' like Abby!"

But even with the acceptance of her peers, school can present certain challenges. "The challenge comes when kids bring special stuff to school for parties and we don't know the exact carb count," Jeanine explains. "Cupcakes can really throw you off!" Jeanine also volunteers to accompany the school on field trips so that Abby can go along.

Abby is a very active seven-year-old, involved in soccer, swimming, and dance classes. Jeanine has had to experiment with the best regime for her during her activities, and has found that Abby does best if she takes her pump off for an hour during a soccer game.

Jeanine recommends that parents who are considering pump therapy for their young children educate themselves as much as possible, and find a health care team that is willing to work patiently with you and your child. Jeanine also feels fortunate that Abby has a twin brother Christopher at school with her, who takes her to the nurse when she feels low and who carries an extra juice box for Abby in his backpack—just in case.

Another "young pumper" success story comes from Noah Levick, who was diagnosed at age three and started pump therapy in first grade. Noah's parents speak of how much their whole family's lifestyle has improved since starting pump therapy. "Not only is Noah's control much better, but our lifestyle is so much better. Noah has a birthday party nearly every weekend, and before he started the pump, it was so hard to explain that he couldn't eat all the cake and ice cream he wanted like other kids. It was tough," Judy Levick describes.

Judy, like Jeanine, is Noah's "pancreas" even when he's at school.

Judy is always reachable by her cell phone. Though she writes down how much insulin to bolus for Noah's lunch, the school nurse calls Judy every day after Noah tests his blood sugar so that Judy can instruct her about how to make any adjustment for a high or low blood sugar. Judy feels that that constant access by cell phone has made Noah's adjustment at school a real success.

Noah is pretty comfortable with the look and feel of the pump. Judy also came to school and read a book to his class so that they could ask questions about diabetes and the pump. "It's really an okay thing to them. Every kid has something, whether it's a peanut allergy or a hearing aid. The kids have been very cool and accepting," she reports.

Judy's found a very good way to make inserting Noah's infusion sets a smooth process—she just puts on a TV show and Noah becomes hypnotized and lets her go about her business. Noah has taken on some of his diabetes management chores himself: He checks his own blood sugar twice a day.

"I would definitely recommend pump therapy to other parents," Judy says. "But remember, you're trading one set of problems for another. With pump therapy, it is much, much more work for Mom and Dad. We check Noah's blood sugar up to ten times per day."

Judy also found a teenage baby-sitter, through the Juvenile Diabetes Research Foundation, who has diabetes herself. Noah loves her, and Judy and her husband can go out, feeling confident that Noah's baby-sitter understands how to deal with high and low blood sugars.

The Levicks also allow Noah to sleep overnight at a friend's house; he just needs to test his blood sugar in the morning and call home to get his breakfast bolus.

As Noah grows, his basal rates need to be adjusted, so the Levicks have gone through many periods of being up during the night to find his correct rates. That is all part of the package for parents who make the commitment to help their kids pump insulin.

As children get older, parents can allow them to take even greater responsibility in their diabetes management—teaching them how to figure out carbohydrate counting and how to determine a bolus of insulin. But even in older children, parents must be on hand for supervision and to correct any errors that children may make.

TEN CONSIDERATIONS

FOR STARTING PUMP THERAPY
FOR YOUR CHILDREN

1. Consider your child's diabetes control—especially if your child experiences severe high or low blood sugars, pump therapy could help even out his or her control.

2. Make sure your commitment is firm. You may have to "work harder" in the sense of testing blood sugar more often, etc.

3. Talk to your child about what the pump looks like and how it will be attached. It's never a good idea to suddenly spring a pump onto a child.

4. Find a doctor and health care team that can support your decision and will work with you.

5. Talk to your child's teachers, school nurse, and administrators about their role in your child's health care. Offer them books and information about pump therapy.

6. Talk to your child's classmates about diabetes and the insulin pump. Answer all of their questions in a straightforward fashion.

7. Talk to your child's friends' parents about how they can help out during play dates, sleepovers, birthday parties, etc.

8. Buy a cell phone and make sure that one parent (or a knowledgeable grandparent, aunt, etc.) is available by phone at all times.

9. Encourage your child to communicate—the more she can express how she feels, the better you can help her.

10. Remember—even with the pump, your child's blood sugars won't be perfect all the time. Don't beat yourself up when your child goes high or low—this is just a reality of life with diabetes.

TWENTY-THREE

Pumping Teens

EACH LIFE STAGE presents unique challenges related to developmental growth. While parents of young children need to be ever vigilant in monitoring their children's diabetes, parents of teenagers need to begin the process of letting go, and allowing their growing children to assume the mantle of responsibilities for their diabetes control. Teenagers can be ideal candidates for pump therapy—their changing schedules and desires to fit in with their friends can make the pump the best solution out there for their diabetes management. But the freedom the pump gives can work successfully only if the teen makes the commitment to the responsibility that the pump also requires.

Jillian Necky is an active fifteen-year-old who was diagnosed with diabetes at age nine. When she first heard about the pump, she thought it sounded cool and really wanted the freedom of not having to worry if she missed a meal and of being able to eat whatever food her friends did when they went to the mall.

Jillian did pretty well with her initial transition. She wore her pump on the belt loop of her jeans, and most kids at school just thought it was a pager. Her friends were cool and casual about her pump, and her best friend would sit with Jillian when she had to test her blood sugar at lunch.

But Jillian also learned that the pump was easy to abuse. She found herself "forgetting" to take a bolus before she ate or to test her blood sugar. When she went to the doctor, he found that she had an A1c of 9.9. Jillian's doctor and parents told her that unless things changed, she'd have to go off the pump.

Jillian decided to take charge of her pump therapy once again, and two months later, her A1c had fallen to 7.8 percent, and she was feeling much better. "It was a real wake-up call," Jillian says.

Now that Jillian is back to careful monitoring, she finds that pump therapy allows her to do absolutely anything other teens do. Recently, she went on an eight-day rafting trip. She took along Ziploc bags for her blood sugar meter and got a waterproof case for her pump, and had a total blast on her rafting excursion. "I could swim with the waterproof case and didn't have to worry if we fell off the raft," she says. "I loved it!" Jillian's parents allowed her the independence of taking that trip because she had proven her ability to manage her diabetes control on her own.

SUCCESS STORIES

Ashley Beard—Pump Enthusiast

HOW DO you get a teen to try the pump? For Ashley Beard, sixteen, her parents dangled a pretty hefty carrot in front of her: Ashley wanted to go on a trip to Europe with her Latin class, and her mom knew that the pump would be the most flexible way for Ashley to control her blood sugars across different time zones, with an erratic schedule, and irregular mealtimes. Mom and Dad said that if she'd try the pump, she could go on the trip. Ashley, who had, in her own words "previously despised the idea of the pump," decided that the trip was worth her trying it.

For the record, the trip was, sadly, canceled, but Ashley has never regretted her decision to go on the pump. "My control has gotten much better, and if I want to go to the mall, I don't need to carry insulin and syringes. It gives you a sense of freedom that I didn't realize was possible," she says. Ashley, who has had diabetes since age three, has had an easy time with her transition to pump therapy, and is active in her high school drama program and swim team.

Ashley hopes to one day travel to Europe, but meanwhile is most happy with her decision to pump, with her newfound freedom and control. She advices other teens to "just try it!" And be sure to pick the pump color you want.

Joe and Jessica, brother and sister, who began pumping when Joe was eleven and Jessica was thirteen, have had a pretty successful run, with some glitches along the way. Doreen, their mom, took charge of most of the kids' pump management during the first six months of their pumping, and then let Joe and Jessica take charge from then on.

Doreen did not have a great experience talking with her kids' teachers and nurses about pump therapy. "They were very negative about the whole thing, until I told them that they didn't have a choice! The pumps were coming," Doreen recalls. The first time the kids went back to school with their pumps, they were stopped by security guards when they entered the school's metal detectors. "The guard wanted to take our pumps away!" Jessica remembers.

Fortunately, both Jessica and Joe felt okay about going on the pump. Jessica had previously experienced bad seizures from low blood sugar, and was willing to try anything to avoid them. "I thought the pump looked cool, and my best friend was really supportive and cool. Everyone at school was pretty interested in it at first and asked me if they could push the buttons for me," she says.

Jessica generally clips her pump onto pants or a skirt and wears a two-piece bathing suit when she swims. She loves eating the food she wants and not having to take shots.

Brother Joe was a little freaked out that the pump would give him too much insulin or that he would mess it up somehow, but those fears have gone away since he's been successfully pumping for three years. He puts his pump in his pants pocket and tucks in the tubing.

Joe has gone into DKA (diabetic ketoacidosis), unfortunately, when his tubing was clogged and the problem was caught too late.

Still, both Jessica and Joe prefer pumping insulin to their old routine, and Mom Doreen agrees that this new method is much preferable to the old way. Doreen deals with the ongoing balance of supervising her kids and allowing them the freedom to start taking care of their diabetes on their own, as they will have to do as adults.

TEN TIPS

FOR TEENS
AND PUMPING

1. Teens who go on pump therapy must be willing to take primary responsibility for their diabetes management.

2. Parents of teens should not abandon their children, but must take a step back in allowing their teens to be the key person in charge.

3. Teen should have an ongoing communication with parents and doctors, and know that they can ask for help at any time.

4. Parents should educate school officials, just as with young children, about management of the pump.

5. Parents must make sure that any adult responsible for the teen—whether leading a field trip, camping excursion, youth group activity, etc. is educated about the pump.

6. Parents should still be reachable by phone at all times.

7. Teens can enjoy the flexibility of eating what their friends eat—as long as they remember to bolus properly to cover the carbs in favorite teen foods, like pizza.

8. Teens can benefit from finding pen pals or other kids on the pump, with whom to "compare notes."

9. Teens can find fashion solutions that make them feel comfortable with wearing the pump.

10. Teens should have a buddy or best friend who can always be there to support them when they're in need.

TWENTY-FOUR

Pumping Seniors

PERHAPS THE GREATEST obstacle to moving more senior citizens from multiple injection to insulin pump therapy is the mistaken belief that you cannot teach older people new things. Sometimes this thinking comes from the medical establishment; at other times it is an internalized feeling expressed by the seniors themselves. Either way, nothing could be further from the truth: senior citizens who make a full commitment to learn pump therapy can succeed just as easily as younger people.

Remember the experience of Mort Waldbaum—Mort had had type 1 diabetes for forty-one years when he made the move to pump therapy, at age seventy-four. For Mort, that meant forty-one years of the same routine of using insulin shots and food exchanges to try to control his diabetes. Even at age seventy-four, when Mort had also gone through a heart attack and bypass surgery, he was not ready to give up and settle for mediocre diabetes care. It was Mort's *desire* for improving his health and his belief that the quality of his life was valuable enough to make a significant change that made him a successful candidate for pump therapy. His age did not impair his ability to learn the mechanics of the pump or learn carb counting or any of the other management skills needed to succeed in pump therapy.

Mort also credits his wife, his main supporter, for helping him succeed with pump therapy. "She is more helpful than you can imagine," Mort says, beaming. "She takes me to all my doctors' appointments, cooks the food that I need to eat, and does whatever needs to be done." Mort and his wife have worked out a system in which Mort eats exactly thirty grams of carbohydrates at each meal, allowing him to keep his fasting blood sugars at 90mg/dL and his post-meal readings at 140.

Dora Roberts, age seventy, has type 2 diabetes, which is most commonly found in people over age forty (although this factor is quickly changing). Like many people with type 2, Dora hoped that she would not have to go on insulin. Type 2 diabetes differs significantly from type 1 in that the pancreas does not make *enough* insulin or the body does not use the insulin that it makes properly, or both. Hence, many people with type 2 are able to treat their diabetes with diet, exercise, and diabetes medication, which lowers blood glucose.

Dora, like many other folks with type 2, was extremely overweight when she was diagnosed, and was first put on diabetes medication. "I was really shocked, although I shouldn't have been," Dora remembers. "Type 2 diabetes was common in my family. My grandmother had had it, and several uncles had it, as well as my brother. I knew I was heavy, but I guess I didn't realize how heavy I was. I had really let my weight problem get the best of me. And then, when I was diagnosed in my early sixties, I thought, 'I'll get rid of this.' So I worked really hard at the weight loss and started on an exercise program."

Dora had great success in her weight-loss efforts: Over the next two years, she dropped eighty-eight pounds and met her goal weight. But her blood sugars were still bouncing up and down. "My doctor kept encouraging me to lose the weight; she thought we'd have an easier time managing my sugars once the weight was off," Dora explains. They experimented with a number of different pills, none bringing about the desired effects. "My sugars were running high most of the time," Dora says. "I'd wake up between 200 and 250, and I just thought, 'Well, I'm diabetic, what else can I do?'"

Dora's doctor was extremely concerned about Dora's control, and saw that Dora had a happy, active life with family, friends, and her church activities, and wanted her to spend her senior years in as good health as possible. Unfortunately, in a routine eye exam, Dora's ophthalmologist found signs of retinopathy, caused by poor blood sugar control, and Dora underwent a series of laser treatments.

"That was it," Dora said. "I told my doctor, 'Give me insulin or whatever it is I need!'" Dora's doctor immediately showed her pictures of the pump and gave her literature about it to take home and think about. Dora made her decision rather quickly.

"I really liked the look of the thing, like a little pager," Dora recalls. "I showed my grandkids the pictures and they told me it looked cool!" Dora was most excited that the pump would easily allow her to continue her walking routine, and held the greatest hope for keeping her blood sugars running even.

Although Dora is a widow who lives alone, she has friends, family, and neighbors next door whom she doesn't hesitate to call if she needs some help. "When I first got started, I had my grandkids help me change the batteries and all of those things until I got the hang of it," Dora recalls. "I did not like those infusion sets, but now I'm an old pro at putting them in."

Most important, Dora's blood sugar control has improved immensely, and she has accepted her diabetes as part of her life. "Maybe if I had been better about my weight before, I wouldn't have to deal with this now," Dora says. "But it is what it is, and I'm thankful I have it under control now."

Whether you (or someone you love) is a senior citizen with type 1 or type 2 diabetes, the insulin pump is a viable option for your diabetes management. In American society, we are seeing people live to unprecedented ages, and people with diabetes should be able to use all the technology available to them to lead a long, happy, and healthy life. The insulin pump can be a tool in making that dream into a reality.

TEN CONSIDERATIONS

FOR SENIOR CITIZENS
WHO WANT TO PUMP

1. Whether you have type 1 or type 2 diabetes, the pump may be a consideration for you.

2. Read all the literature available about the insulin pump, and show your doctor that you are knowledgeable.

3. Find a health care team who will support your decision—even if it means leaving a doctor you've worked with for years.

4. Enlist family members or friends to help support your decision.

5. Be patient with yourself—switching to pump therapy means a lot of new learning for everyone.

6. Join an insulin pump support group and learn from experienced pump users.

7. If there are certain parts of the mechanics of pump therapy that are hard for you to work with, ask your diabetes educator, a friend, or support person to work with you on that task until you feel comfortable.

8. Continue to be active—pump therapy can work well with your fitness regime.

9. If you are on Medicare, remember that your pump company will deal directly with Medicare agents so you don't have to waste time getting caught up in their "red tape."

10. Be an inspiration to others—tell other senior citizens about how the pump has improved the quality of your life!

TWENTY-FIVE

Pumping and Pregnancy

IN HER LANDMARK study "Continuous Subcuta-neous Insulin Infusion (CSII) Therapy During Pregnancy," Donna L. Jornsay, RN, BSN, CPNP, CDE, finds that CSII (insulin pump therapy) offers distinct advantages for pregnant women. Insulin pump therapy mimics normal physiology of the pancreas, allowing for tighter blood sugar control; it allows the pregnant woman to adjust her basal rates with the varying insulin requirements that go along with different stages of pregnancy; it allows for management of morning sickness; it allows for increased flexibility both during pregnancy and postpartum; it allows for a decrease in glucose excursion, reductions in hypoglycemia, and less DKA.

All of these factors are critical for pregnant women because high blood glucose levels in a pregnant woman can lead to birth defects in the baby as well as serious health risks for the expecting mother. Blood glucose goals during pregnancy are: fasting, 60 to 90 mg/dL, pre-meal values 60 to 100 mg/dL, one-hour post-meal values 90 to 120 mg/dL, and middle-of-the-night values 70 to 120 mg/dL. These strict goals may seem daunting, but fortunately, pump therapy allows a woman the easiest means out there to achieve them.

Jornsay does not have experience with insulin pump therapy only as a clinician; she also has firsthand life experience as a person living with type 1 diabetes who used pump therapy for over twenty years and has successfully carried and delivered two healthy daughters.

"I've been on the pump for twenty-two years," Donna Jornsay explains. "I stuck with it through the early days, when it was so big that you couldn't wear it on anything elastic and everything you wore had to have a belt, because I felt so much better when I was on it and could keep my blood sugars in control." Donna was a sort of experiment with pump therapy and pregnancy during her own two pregnancies; when she went into the hospitals, none of the health care workers understood the pump, and wanted to get her on NPH insulin immediately! "I had to be savvy enough to convince them to let me stay on the pump," Donna explains.

Over time, Donna, a registered nurse and certified diabetes educator, used her personal success to help other women with diabetes by running a diabetes and pregnancy program. Donna is convinced, through the experience of working with so many women, that pump therapy is the best way to insure a healthy delivery for both baby and mom. Donna was kind enough to help me understand the findings of her study and to put them in layperson's terms.

To begin with, pump therapy, for everyone, has been proven to cause less blood sugar fluctuation and so improve overall control and lower A1cs. For pregnant women (and women trying to conceive) this factor is critical. Donna breaks down the varying insulin requirements during pregnancy this way: During the first trimester, many women experience an increased need for insulin, much as they might during the premenstrual phase of their monthly cycle. From weeks nine to sixteen of pregnancy, insulin requirements suddenly drop, causing many women to experience severe hypoglycemia, often with them not being able to feel their usual symptoms. From week sixteen on, insulin requirements slowly increase from week to week. At the very end of pregnancy, insulin requirement may drastically drop off again.

Pump therapy allows the patient (with medical supervision, of course) to make all the adjustments needed to balance those fluctuations through the adjustment of basal rates. The pump alone can deliver the precise amounts of insulin needed to sustain a woman's blood sugar control during the night and early morning hours without putting her in danger of getting low blood sugar.

Donna also notes how important pump therapy is for women who experience morning sickness. "If you are feeling nauseous and are concerned that the nausea may progress to vomiting, we recommend that you take part of your pre-meal bolus. If you can tolerate the food and have no trouble keeping it down, then you can take the rest of your bolus and eat the rest of your meal," she explains. The advice may sound simple, but for women dealing with ongoing bouts of nausea, this flexibility can make all the difference in maintaining blood sugar goals.

Donna recommends that women who want to get pregnant get on the pump before trying to conceive, and work with their health care team to achieve good blood sugar control. Because blood sugar control is critical during the first few weeks after conception, when important developmental stages are occurring in the fetus, a pregnant woman should strive for excellent control from the start. But if you are pregnant now and have not yet started pump therapy, don't despair: Women can be successfully educated and adjusted to the pump during any stage of pregnancy. Pregnant women selecting pump therapy *must* regularly monitor blood glucose and learn to match insulin boluses with carbohydrate counting. They must also be willing to keep all of their medical appointments and commit to working closely with their health care providers. Several other factors necessary to carry a healthy baby should be considered before trying to conceive. If you are not an ideal body weight, try to lose weight; if you smoke, you must quit before trying to conceive; if you drink caffeine, cut down to one cup of coffee (or one soft drink) per day; if you aren't regularly exercising, get into an established fitness routine; and also, begin taking folic acid, which prevents birth defects. It is important to remember that it takes the average American woman at least five months to actually get pregnant, fertility is not increased or decreased by diabetes. However, women with poor blood sugar control will not be able to successfully carry a baby through the first trimester.

It is critical that a woman find an obstetrician who is experienced in working with women with diabetes. The doctor should be someone whom you feel comfortable talking with and asking any questions of. You should also make sure that the hospital at which you plan to deliver is equipped with a level II neonatal intensive care unit, should any problems in the baby arise. "Talk to your doctor ahead of time about what your hospital's policies are," Donna suggests. "Many hospitals routinely place a baby from a diabetic mom in the nursery for six hours after the birth, to monitor blood sugars. If you know this ahead of time, it won't be so upsetting as finding out right after delivery."

Another important point for any pregnant woman with diabetes to know is that it's critical to check your morning urine for ketones, which can cause damage to your baby. Ketones are caused when the body breaks down fat, and in pregnant women this can occur when a woman hasn't eaten in nine to twelve hours. Donna recommends that women take a small snack of protein before bed to prevent the occurrence of ketones.

At about twenty-six weeks, women will need to move their infusion site away from the abdomen to somewhere else that has an inch of so of fat—the hips, thighs, or arms work well. It is also critical that women change infusion sites every two days during pregnancy to insure against a problem with insulin absorption.

"When you pack your bags for the hospital, take along plenty of pump supplies and your own blood glucose monitor," Donna warns. During labor and delivery, your blood sugar will be monitored every hour, and you may not need any insulin at all. Many women keep their pump connected, running on suspend; that way, if they do need to take a bolus, it is convenient to do so. Many women find that they need no insulin at all for the day or two following delivery. Keeping your pump connected can also be advantageous during a cesarean birth and following it—especially as many women who experience cesareans can take in only small amounts of food for the first few days afterward.

Pump therapy is also a great aid in the postpartum stage, especially for women who are breastfeeding. It is important to keep blood sugar control tight during breastfeeding, as excess glucose could be transmitted to the baby. The stressful routine of being a new mother can be improved by making adjustments in your pump therapy—if you have to skip a meal or find yourself sleeping at odd intervals, your basal rates can help you maintain good blood sugar control.

Today's technology allows for women with diabetes, who are motivated and properly educated, to carry and deliver a healthy baby, with no complications for mother or child. Being pregnant for a woman with diabetes requires hard work and commitment, but insulin pump therapy offers her the best way possible to achieve the dream of a complication-free pregnancy.

TEN TIPS
for Moms-to-Be

1. If you are not on pump therapy already, talk to your health care team immediately about making the move.

2. Wait at least three months once you start pump therapy to get adjusted, before you start trying to conceive.

3. If you are already on the pump, make sure that you are in the best control possible—work with your doctor, educator, and/or nutritionist to achieve optimal control.

4. Make sure that you take care of any other issues that could affect the health of your baby: Stop smoking, cut down caffeine, get into an exercise routine, reach your ideal weight, and take folic acid.

5. Find both an obstetrician who specializes in the care of women with diabetes and an endocrinologist who is experienced in caring for pregnant women with diabetes.

6. Make sure that the hospital where you plan to deliver has at least a level III neonatal intensive care unit.

7. Keep your blood sugars in as tight control as possible. Pregnancy goals are: fasting, 60 to 90 mg/dL, pre-meal values 60 to 100 mg/dL, one-hour post-meal values 90 to 120 mg/dL, and middle-of-the-night values 70 to 120 mg/dL.

8. Remember—no one can reach those goals all the time! Do your very best, but don't beat yourself up when you occasionally fall short.

9. Find support—a support group with other pregnant women with diabetes can help you keep perspective and allow you to compare notes with others facing the same challenges.

10. Stay active, relaxed, and healthy! Rest as needed, eat balanced foods, try prenatal yoga. The healthier you are during pregnancy, the better your chances that your baby will be healthy and strong.

What Lies Ahead in Insulin Pump Technology

IT IS TRULY awesome to consider the advances in technology that have so dramatically improved the quality of diabetes care during the last twenty years. The insulin pump has, of course, been at the center of technology. To remember what the pump looked like when it was first introduced and to compare those old-fashioned models with one of today's pumps shows us that technology truly holds the possibility for improving the quality of diabetes care. Much research is currently being conducted to take today's pumps and improve them to the next level. If we can only keep our blood sugars in as good control as possible now, it seems clear that tools will be coming along in the near future that will be able to enhance our control.

Some of the most exciting research is being funded by Medtronic MiniMed and Disetronic. One new product that Medtronic MiniMed currently has on the market is an external glucose sensor. It looks something like a pump, and is available through Medtronic MiniMed. You wear the external sensor like a pump for approximately three days, and record everything that you eat during that time. The sensor will then provide you with data that with your physician's help, you will be able to analyze to understand exactly how different food items affect your blood sugar. In other words, you will have information about what is going on with your blood sugar in between regular blood sugar testing.

Medtronic MiniMed is also working on a combination of their sensor with the insulin pump. In other words, these would be long-term sensors that work in conjunction with the pump, to determine insulin needs based on blood sugar results. Research on this implantable pump-sensor combination is currently in progress; for more detailed information, check out Medtronic MiniMed's Web site at www.minimed.com.

Disetronic, whose company headquarters are based in Switzerland, is working on some other exciting technological advances.

For one thing, they have a product that has been approved on the market in Europe for people who have trouble with infusion sites. Called the Diaport, it is a small implanted metal ball that requires less insulin and more predictable absorption. It will take some time for the Diaport to be fully approved for use in the United States. To learn more about Diaport, you can log on to the Disetronic page at www.disatronic-usa.com/products/diaport.htm.

Disetronic is also working on the semi-closed loop system called ADICOL that is in its third year of research in Europe. ADICOL is a prototype pancreas that delivers insulin continuously under the skin and maintains blood sugar, or glucose, at a constant level.

The prototype is made up of three parts: a sensor placed on the skin that measures blood glucose levels, a hand-held computer that analyses this information, and a small pump that infuses insulin into the body.

With research funded by the European Commission as well as insulin pump manufacturer Disetronic, it looks hopeful that ADI-COL will be approved for use in Europe within five years. However, that does mean a longer delay for its approval in the United States, where clinical trials have not begun. To learn more, visit ADICOL's Web site at www.adicol.org.

Both pump companies give us, the pump users, hope that just around the corner, our health care is going to take another tremendous leap forward. For people living with diabetes today, there has never been more hope that we can lead full, healthy, productive lives. May your own journey seeking out the best diabetes management possible lead you to a life of healthy choices for you as a whole person, and may diabetes never stop you from reaching and living your dreams.

GLOSSARY OF DIABETES AND INSULIN PUMP TERMS

BASAL INSULIN—In insulin pump therapy, basal insulin is the *baseline* continual delivery of small amounts of insulin.

BOLUS INSULIN—Additional insulin given before eating to cover the carbohydrates in the food about to be ingested.

CANNULA—This is the small plastic tube at the end of the infusion set. It is inserted just under the skin using a small needle. Insulin is delivered through the cannula into the fatty tissue in your abdomen (or wherever your insert it).

CARBOHYDRATES—A part of food that includes fiber, sugars, and starches. Starch is created from energy from the sun, carbon dioxide and water. Glucose, a single sugar, is the building block of starch. Carbohydrates mainly come from plant food, like grains, fruits, and vegetables, and also from milk products.

CSII—Continuous subcutaneous insulin infusion, another name for insulin pump therapy, commonly found in medical literature.

DAWN PHENOMENON—a condition in which blood sugar rises during the early morning hours.

DIABETIC KETOACIDOSIS (DKA)—a condition in which ketones are present in the body, and if not treated, can lead to sickness, coma, or even death. This condition is caused when a person with diabetes does not receive the proper amount of insulin.

ENDOCRINOLOGIST—physician specializing in the treatment of the endocrine glands and their secretions, which includes the treatment of diabetes.

GLUCAGON—A hormone that stimulates the liver to release glucose into the blood. People with diabetes should carry a *glucagon kit* that allows a person to inject glucagon directly into the bloodstream, in the case of extreme hypoglycemia.

GLYCEMIC INDEX—a ranking of foods based on their immediate effect on blood sugar levels.

GLYCOGEN—Excess sugar in the body becomes converted into glycogen and is stored in the liver.

HEMOGLOBIN A1c (A1c)—a blood test that reflects average blood glucose levels during the previous 60 to 90 days. Used by clinicians, along with daily blood glucose logs, to monitor diabetes control.

HYPERGLYCEMIA—high blood glucose; can be characterized by hunger, thirst, frequent urination, upset stomach, dry skin, fruity smell on breath, blurry vision, and headache.

HYPOGLYCEMIA—low blood glucose; can be characterized by confusion, sleepiness, irritability, fatigue, weakness, dizziness, sweating, shakiness, and pale skin.

KETONES—waste products that are made when the body turns stored fat into energy.

INSULIN PUMP—a battery-powered, computerized device approximately the size of a pager that delivers insulin through tubing that is connected to a needle or catheter placed under the skin.

INFUSION SET—a metal insertion needle pushes a tiny, flexible plastic tube under the skin. The tubing connects the pump to the pump wearer.

TYPE 1 DIABETES—most often occurring in people under age thirty, the body stops making insulin or makes only a minute amount. Most likely caused when the body's auto-antibodies attack insulin or the cells that make insulin.

TYPE 2 DIABETES—most often occurring in people over age forty, the body does not make enough insulin or has trouble using what insulin it makes. Type 2 runs in families and can be brought on as a result of obesity.

COUNTING CARBOHYDRATES

WHY COUNT CARBOHYDRATES?

The chart below illustrates the importance of counting carbohydrates to determine bolus insulin needs. Ninety to 100 percent of all carbohydrates that we eat are converted into glucose; some carbs convert in just 15 to 30 minutes, while others takes a longer time to be absorbed into the bloodstream (gradually over 60 to 90 minutes). Because the insulin pump relies on fast-acting insulin, the pumper needs to bolus the correct amount of insulin to cover all carbohydrates that are eaten. A small amount of fats are also converted into glucose, while most of the fats transform into glycerol and fatty acids, which the body then stores as fat.

	APPROXIMATE AMOUNT CONVERTED TO GLUCOSE	TIME UNTIL GLUCOSE PEAKS
Carbohydrates	90–100 percent	Simple carbs: 15–30 mins. Complex: 60–90 mins.
Fat	<10 percent	Several Hours

DETERMINING BOLUS INSULIN BASED ON CARBOHYDRATE COUNTING

The following table provides a sample breakdown of how to determine bolus insulin for a sample snack.

*Note: Most adults with Type One diabetes need 1 unit of fast-acting insulin for every 10 to 15 grams of carbohydrates, but individuals may need more or less than 1 unit. Your doctor or diabetes educator will help you to determine how much insulin you need for every 10–15 grams of carbohydrate. The following sample calculation is based on the 1 unit theory.

FOOD	GRAMS OF CARB PER SERVING	X SERVINGS	= TOTAL CARBS
Apple	19	2	38
Yogurt (6 oz. light)	16	1	16
Total carbs for this meal:			54

Estimated carb ratio: 1 unit for every twelve grams of carbohydrates

Total grams carbohydrates *54* divided by carb ratio *12* = 4.6 units of insulin

REFERENCES

Cersosimo, Eugene, M.D., Ph.D. *Improved Clinical Outcomes with Intensive Insulin Pump Therapy in Type 1 Diabetes.* San Francisco, June 2002.

Colberg, Sheri R., Ph.D. and John Walsh, PA, CDE. "Pumping Insulin During Exercise: What Healthcare Providers and Diabetic Patients Need to Know," *The Physician and Sports Medicine.* April 2002.

Foster-Powell, Kaye, M. Nutr. & Diet., Jennie Brand-Miller, Ph.D., Stephen Colagiuri, M.D., and Thomas Wolever, M.S. *The Glucose Revolution.* New York: Marlowe & Company, 1999.

Foster-Powell, Kaye, M. Nutr. & Diet., Jennie Brand-Miller, Ph.D., Stephen Colagiuri, M.D., Thomas Wolever, M.S. *The Glucose Revolution Pocket Guide to Diabetes.* New York: Marlowe & Company, 2000.

Foster-Powell, Kaye, M. Nutr. & Diet., Susannah Holt, and Janette Brand-Miller, Ph.D. "International table of glycemic index and glycemic load values: 2002," *American Journal of Clinical Nutrition.* July 2002.

Freemark, Michael, M.D. "Effective Insulin Pump Therapy for Infants and Young Children with Type 1 Diabetes," *Journal of Pediatrics.* September 2002.

Hanaire-Broutin, H., M.D. "Comparison of CSII and multiple injection regimes using insulin lispro in type 1 diabetic patients on intensified treatment: a randomized study," *Diabetes Care.* September 2000.

Jornsay, Donna L., RN, BSN, CPNP, CDE. "Continuous Subcutaneous Insulin Infusion (CSII) Therapy During Pregnancy." *Diabetes Spectrum, Vol. 11, No. 1,* 1998.

Kamoi, Kyuzi, M.D. "Good Long-Term Quality of Life Without Diabetic Complications with 20 Years of Continuous Subcutaneous Insulin Infusion Therapy in a Brittle Diabetic Elderly Patient," *Diabetes Care.* February 2002.

King, Allen B., M.D. *Basal Insulin: Continuous Glucose Monitoring Reveals Less Overnight Hypoglycemia with Continuous Subcutaneous Insulin Infusion than with Glargine.* San Francisco, June 2002.

Pennington, Jean A. T. *Bowes & Church's Food Values of Portions Commonly Used.* Philadelphia: Lippincott-Raven Publishers, 1998.

Pickup, John, DCPHIL, FRCPATH and Harry Keen, CBE, M.D., FRCP. "Continuous Subcutaneous Insulin Infusion at 25 Years," *Diabetes Care.* March 2002.

Pozzilli, Paolo. *CSII Versus Intensive Insulin Therapy at Onset of Type 1 Diabetes: The IMDIAB 8 Two-Year Randomized Trials.* San Francisco, June 2002.

Unger, Jeff, M.D. "Case Study: A 62-Year-Old Man with "Brittle" Type 1 Diabetes." *Clinical Diabetes.* Vol. 20, No. 1, 2002.

ACKNOWLEDGMENTS

I FEEL A deep sense of gratitude toward so many people for their personal support of my decision to choose pump therapy, as well as their support of my decision to chronicle my experiences, and those of other pump users, in this book. That constant support fueled my efforts to write a book about the challenges and rewards of insulin pump therapy from a patient's perspective—a book that I couldn't find on any shelf when I was making my own decision to choose the pump.

My thanks go to my endocrinologist, Dr. Ned Weiss, who introduced me to and encouraged me to consider the benefits of insulin pump therapy. My thanks also go to Pam Ladds, MSW, who helped me to realize that I truly could take control over my diabetes, and who encouraged me, from day one, to write this book.

I am grateful to the various professionals in the field of diabetes education and pump therapy who took time out of their busy schedules to help me with this book. My thanks go to Audrey Finkelstein; Linda "Freddi" Fredrickson, MA, RN, CDE; Michael Freemark, M.D.; Donna Jornsay, RN, BSN, CPNP, CDE, Rem Laan; and Gary Schiener, MS CDE. Gary and Freddi were two of my very thorough proofreaders, along with Jessi Nissim and Joellyn Wallen Zollman. I am thankful to each one of you for your careful reading and important feedback. Freddi also helped me tremendously by sharing invaluable articles and resources about pump therapy. Special thanks go to my sister, Julie Kaplan Borenstein, Ph.D., for her insight and guidance about issues dealing with diabetes, depression, and mental illness.

This book would not have been possible without the many willing people who were so generous in taking time to talk with me about their experiences with insulin pump therapy. Although I was not able to use everyone's story in the final version of the book, each person's interview had a great impact on my writing and affected the content of this book. I am grateful to have found so many folks who spoke openly and honestly about how pump therapy has shaped their experience with their diabetes, and every aspect of their lives.

My deepest thanks go to Matthew Lore, publisher of Marlowe & Company, who truly understood my vision for this book and has shown me continual support in the process of writing it. Matthew, who himself has type 1 diabetes, got started on insulin pump therapy while I was working on this manuscript. I am most appreciative that Marlowe & Company is publishing the "demystified" series of health-related books—a most needed addition for patients and professionals alike.

Many of my dear friends and family members offered me encouragement in writing this book—from brainstorming about my initial vision to helping me connect with people to interview. My brother, Jon Kaplan, read the very earliest draft of my manuscript and encouraged me to go on. Special thanks go to my husband, Fred Kaplan-Mayer, for loving and encouraging me in all of my creative pursuits.

INDEX

A

adhesive tape, allergy to, 135
ADICOL (Disetronic), 177
adrenaline, 141
air bubbles, 124
airports and security, 148-150
alarms, on pump, 51, 53, 72, 75
alcohol, 110
allergic reactions, to infusion sets, 135
Altman, Yerachmiel (profile), 11-12,
    48, 72, 122, 128, 135, 138
American Association of Diabetes
    Educators, 22
American Diabetes Association
    financial assistance for pump
        users, 63
    referrals to endocrinologist, 16
    Web site, 22
Animas, 18, 22, 64
Animas R-1000, 94-95
anxiety, therapy for, 28-29
Asian foods, 108
athletics. *see* exercise issues

B

baby-sitters, 159
bagels, 106-107
basal insulin
    adjusting for exercise, 10, 76-78

changes through childhood, 159
defined, 10, 179
first setting, 113-115
nighttime levels, 53, 114
record-keeping, 79
and stress, 140-141
and travel across time zones,
    150-151
and weight loss, 128-129
basketball, 81
bathing suits, 85
batteries, 33, 35, 53, 66, 123-124
beaches, 85-86
Beard, Ashley (profile), 162-163
bleeding, at insertion site, 134-135
blood glucose. *see* blood sugar
blood sugar
    dawn phenomenon, 3, 179
    low, after sex, 57
blood sugar control
    and birth defects, 170-171
    easier using pump, 31-32
    and exercise, 76-77
    and impotence, 57, 59
    and pregnancy, 173
blood sugar logs, 65
blood sugar testing
    before and after sex, 55, 57-58,
    59

before bed, 53
more diligence needed with
    pump, 32, 83
nighttime, 35, 53
body image concerns, 39-40, 55
bolus insulin/bolusing
    calculating, 103-104
    carbohydrate counting to
        determine, 103, 180-181
    children, 52, 157-158, 160
    defined, 10, 179
    and fruits and vegetables, 105
    learning to use, 114-115
    limits, with pump, 72
    and morning sickness, 172
    at restaurants, 108
books, online, 22
*Bowes & Church's Food Values of
    Portions Commonly Used,* 104
bras, 49
breastfeeding, 174

C
cannula, 179
carbohydrate counting
    calculating, 104-105
    carbohydrates defined, 179
    committing to, 35
    determining bolus based on, 103,
        180-181
    exchange system, 102
    and glycemic index, 106-107
    health benefits of, 110
cell phones, for parents, 159, 160
cesarean births, 173
children
    birthday parties, 107
    carbohydrate counting, 105, 107
    carrying supplies, 67
    changing infusion sites, 132, 133
    commitment by parents needed,
        33
    emotional issues, 138
    finding out about diabetes, 1-2

preschoolers, 155-156
and pump mechanics, 73
at school, 157-158, 160
sleepovers, 52
and sports, 158
swimming pool activity and, 87
toddlers, 155-156
Chinese foods, 108
Chub, Joyce, 71
church support groups, 28
clothing, and pump visibility, 40-43,
    45-47, 85
Cohen, David (profile), 51, 55, 86,
    109, 122, 134
commitments, necessary to succeed,
    31-35
conception, attempting, 172-173
contact sports, 81
CSII (Continuous subcutaneous
    insulin infusion), 179

D
DANA (Sooil), 18, 22
dawn phenomenon, 3, 179
Demba, Ernie (profile), 15, 32, 146
Demba, Liessa (profile), 15-16, 46,
    103, 115, 146
Depinto, Sue (profile), 25
depression
    and diabetes, 137-140
    therapy for, 28-29
diabetes
    and depression, 137-140
    public awareness of, 46
    type 1, 180
    type 2, 167, 180
Diabetes, Exercise and Sports
    Association, 22, 77
diabetes educators, finding, 17
diabetes magazines, 21
diabetic ketoacidosis (DKA), 179
Diaport (Disetronic), 177
diet, on pump, 126-130
Disetronic, 18, 22, 61, 64, 177

Disetronic D-Tron pump, 96-97
Disetronic H-Tron Plus pump, 64, 97-98
Doreen (parent), 12, 163-164

E
EMLA cream, 133
emotional health, 137-142
emotional support. *see* pump support groups
endocrinologists, 15-17, 179
exercise issues, 76-83

F
families. *see also* parents
    diabetes and, 138
    support from, 25, 27, 167
fat foods, high-, 109
financial assistance, for pump users, 63
foods
    and bolusing, 104, 105, 108-110
    diet changes with pumping, 126-130
football, 81
Freemark, Michael, 155
friends, support from, 25, 27-28, 144
fruits and vegetables, 104, 105

G
glucagon, 180
The Glucose Revolution Pocket Guide to Diabetes, 107
glucose sensors, external, 176-177
glucose tabs, 53, 78, 83
glycagon kits, 68
glycemic index, 22, 106-107, 180
glycogen, 180

H
health insurance issues, 60-65, 113
heat, exposure to, 86
hemoglobin A1c, 180

hospitalization, for pump transition, 112-117
hyperglycemia, 180
hypoglycemia, 83, 180

I
illness, society's views of, 28-29
impotence, 57
infections, 131-132
infusion sets, 66, 84, 132-133, 180
infusion sites, 49, 74, 82, 131-136, 173
injection therapy, number using, 9
insertion sites. *see* infusion sites
insulin
    FAA security guidelines for traveling with, 148-149
    requirements during pregnancy, 171-172
    shelf life of, 68
    sun-damaged, 86
insulin cartridges, 33, 35, 51, 66
insulin pump models, compared, 94-101
insulin pump therapy
    choosing, 4
    clinical trials, 5, 10-11
    commitments needed, 30-35
    first days on, 112-117
    first weeks on, 121-125
    information sources for
        endocrinologists, 15
        list of, 21
        pump support groups, 19-20, 75
        speaking to other users, 18-20
        Web sites, 16, 18, 22-23
    preparing to start, 89-90
    weight gain with, 126-127
    why switch to?, 11-13
insulin pumps
    about, 9-11, 180
    accessory catalogues, 49
    awareness of wearing, 47-48

back-up plans, 67–68
choosing, 91–93
costs, 60
disconnecting for sex, 55, 56, 58, 59
future developments, 176–178
manuals, 124
manufacturers, 18, 61, 64, 73–74, 92, 123–124
mechanics of, 71–75
monthly supplies, 62–63
size, 9, 10
supplies to carry, 66–70
training, 73–74
upgrading, 63
warranties, 64
insurance. *see* health insurance issues
insurance, property, 60
International Diabetes Federation, 22
Internet. *see* Web sites

J

Jennings, Cara (profile), 42, 104, 134–135, 139–140, 144
Jessica (profile), 163–164
job changes, 62
Joe (profile), 163–164
Johnson, Nicole (profile), 39–40, 43–45
Jornsay, Donna (profile), 170–173
Juvenile Diabetes Research Foundation
    financial assistance for pump users, 63
    referrals to endocrinologist, 16
    Web site, 23

K

Kaplan-Mayer, Gabrielle (profile), 41, 78
ketones, 180
    checking, 35, 82
Kochan, Kathy (profile), 19, 27, 41, 61, 77–78, 105, 127–128, 151

L

Ladds, Pam, 28
Levick, Judy (parent), 158–159
Levick, Noah (profile), 158–159
Lions Club, 63
list serve (online discussion list), 18, 91
Living with Diabetes (Johnson), 43
logs, blood sugar, 65
Lore, Abigail (profile), 156–158
Lore, Jeanine (parent), 156–158
Lore, Matthew (profile), 78–79, 79–80, 121, 151

M

managed health care, 60–65
manuals, pump, 124
Medic Alert tags, 69
Medicaid, 65
medical tags, 69
Medicare, 61, 65
Medtronic MiniMed, 18, 23, 61, 176–177
Medtronic MiniMed 508, 98–99
Medtronic MiniMed Paradigm, 99–101
menstrual cycle, changes around, 3, 122
mental illnesses, 140
metal detectors, 149–150
morning sickness, 170, 172
motivation issues, 143–147

N

National Institutes of Health, 23
Necky, Jillian (profile), 161–162
"nighttime buddy," 116, 117
nutrition guides, 104

P

pajamas, 51, 53
pancreas, function of, 10
parents. *see also* children; teenagers
    availability of, 158–159
    breaks from care for, 144–145

carbohydrate counting, 105
commitment to pump therapy, 33
profiles of success, 156–159, 163–164
and teens on prom night, 42–43
pets, 52, 53
physicians
knowledge of pump therapy, 6, 16, 69
letter from, describing condition, 149
recommendations for specific pump, 91–92
pregnancy, 170–175
premenstrual symptoms, 3
preschoolers, 155–156
Price, Carys (profile), 11, 62, 77, 85, 116, 141
Pritikin diet, 128
psychotherapy. *see* therapy, for depression and anxiety
pump support groups
finding, 19–20, 25, 28
learning from, 75
staying motivated, 144, 147
teenagers, 26
ten reasons to seek, 30
and therapy, 28–29
using in first weeks, 123–124
pump therapy. *see* insulin pump therapy
"Pumping Insulin During Exercise," 76
Pumping Insulin (Walsh), 4

R
record-keeping, 65, 79
Roberts, Dora (profile), 167–168
Rotary Club, 63
Russell, Gary, 73, 106

S
sand, and pump, 85–86
Scheiner, Gary, 17, 72
schools, 157–158, 160

Seeley, Kim (profile), 12, 31, 46, 77, 80–81, 85, 122, 144
Seifert, Sonia (profile), 17, 26, 40, 72
senior citizens, 166–169
sex, 54–59
sleeping, 49–53
Sooil (DANA), 18, 22, 23
Sooil (DANA) Diabecare II, 95–96
stress, coping with, 140–141
S.U.G.A.R. (Canada), 63
sunburns, 86
supplies to carry, for pumps, 66–70
support groups. *see* pump support groups
sweating, and insertion sites, 82, 133–134
Swenson, Judy (profile), 42, 51–52, 138–139
swimming, 84–88

T
teenagers. *see also* parents
carrying supplies, 67
dating, 56
and depression, 139
prom night, 42–43
success profiles, 161–164
support groups for, 26
tips for, 165
temperature extremes, 82, 86
therapy, for depression and anxiety, 28–29
toddlers, 155–156
transitioning, to pumping, 112–117
traveling
FAA security guidelines, 148–149
meals while, 107–108
tubing
air bubbles in, 124
and sleeping, 52

U
United Kingdom, 62

V

vacations, activity during, 151
videos, 75
visibility, of pump, 45–47, 49

W

Waldbaum, Mort (profile), 12, 15, 62, 166–167
water sports and issues, 84–88
Web sites. *see also* list serve (online discussion lists)

general information, 16, 18, 22–23, 77
glycemic index, 107
pump manufacturers', 18, 92
wedding dresses, 41–42
weight–lifting, 77
weight management, 126–130, 167
Weiss, Ned, 78, 113

Y

yoga, 79